Carefree Carnivore Diet For Beginners

Unlock Ancestral Secrets to Lose Fat, Boost Energy, Conquer Inflammation, and Thrive

by Marsha Shepherd Whitt

No Bull Just Publishing / Marsha Shepherd Whitt
Medway, Ohio, USA

ISBN 978-1-966942-00-9

Library of Congress Control Number: 2025901553

Cover images adapted from Chil Veraa, Coco Zinvaa, Rudy & Peter Skitterians, and Presert Taosiri, from Pixabay.com.

Cover design and formatting by No Bull Just Publishing,
https://NoBullJustPublishing.com

NOTE: Although this book includes recipes, and access to online recipe resources, it is not meant to be a "cookbook" therefore it does not contain entertaining images, and is printed in black and white to save on print costs, therefore saving you money.
You're welcome.

I want to express my heartfelt gratitude for choosing this book as your guide. Writing it has been a labor of love, driven by my passion for helping people lead healthier lives. Each page was written with empathy and understanding, acknowledging the challenges and triumphs that come with any lifestyle change. After reading this book, I would be so appreciative if you would consider leaving a review on Amazon, which will help others in need more easily find it. Just click the link below or scan the QR code. Thanks so much!

https://www.amazon.com/review/create-review/?channel=glance-detail&asin=1966942001&ie=UTF8

Introduction

A few years back, I found myself standing in front of the mirror, facing a reflection that didn't match how I felt inside. Managing Hashimoto's Hypothyroidism for decades had left my energy levels low, and I just wasn't myself. It was during this time that my husband, Kevin, stumbled upon the carnivore diet. At first, it seemed like a drastic shift, but the promise of renewed vitality and health was too compelling to ignore. Kevin was all-in from the get-go, but it took me another year to come around. We discovered a path that radically transformed our lives.

This book serves as a reliable, science-backed guide for those new to the carnivore diet. My goal is to dispel common myths and offer structured guidance, enhancing your confidence as you explore this dietary lifestyle.

Allow me to introduce myself. I'm Marsha Shepherd Whitt, an author deeply passionate about health and wellness. My focus has always been on empowering individuals—particularly women and seniors—to achieve their health goals. Through personal experience with the ketogenic and carnivore ways of eating, and high-intensity strength training, Kevin and I have discovered the profound benefits of an ancestral diet.

One thing Kevin helped me to realize is there is a vast difference between 'weight loss' and 'fat loss.' Weight loss might sound appealing, but it often involves losing muscle and bone mass, not just fat. Fat loss, on the other hand, is a different game. It is about feeding your body nutrient-dense foods that keep you strong and satisfied. The carnivore diet excels here by eliminating antinutrients and focusing on real, wholesome nutrition.

The health benefits of the carnivore diet are impressive. Many people report fat loss, a surge in energy, and better management of chronic illnesses. This isn't just anecdotal; experts like Dr. Ken Berry and Dr. Paul Mason, along with several recent studies, support these claims. Throughout this book, you'll find evidence-based content to guide you. But don't just take my word for it; there are scientific and other notations in the References and Endnotes at the back of the book. *Make sure to visit the References and Endnotes and the links provided*.

Of course, there are concerns and misconceptions about this way of eating. Questions about nutrient sufficiency and how to handle social situations often arise. Rest assured, we'll address these issues head-on. You'll find practical advice and tips that make transitioning to this lifestyle both 'feastible' (see what I did there?) and enjoyable.

What sets this book apart is its unique features. It has 60 days of meal plans designed to simplify your journey. We've included access to diverse recipes, make-ahead instruction, meal prep for busy days, and tips for navigating social events without compromising your commitment. You'll also find expert insights and personal success stories to inspire and inform you along the way.

Many of the links in this book, such as for recipes, tips, and personal stories, are to YouTube videos. If you don't have a Google/YouTube account, you can still enjoy all the content in guest mode without having to sign in. Just click the video link, or scan the QR code, sit back, and enjoy.

I invite you to approach this book and the carnivore lifestyle with a radically-open mind, allowing your preconceived notions about diet and nutrition to be challenged. The carnivore diet might be unlike anything you've tried before, but it offers a new perspective on health that's worth exploring.

As you turn these pages, expect to gain actionable steps, structured guidance, and a supportive framework to help you transition into the carnivore diet, including the WHAT, WHY, HOW, WHERE & WHEN to carnivore. This book is a companion on your journey towards improved health and vitality.

I'm genuinely excited to share this knowledge with you. My commitment is to support you every step of the way. Let's embark on this transformative journey together. Your path to better health starts now.

WHAT

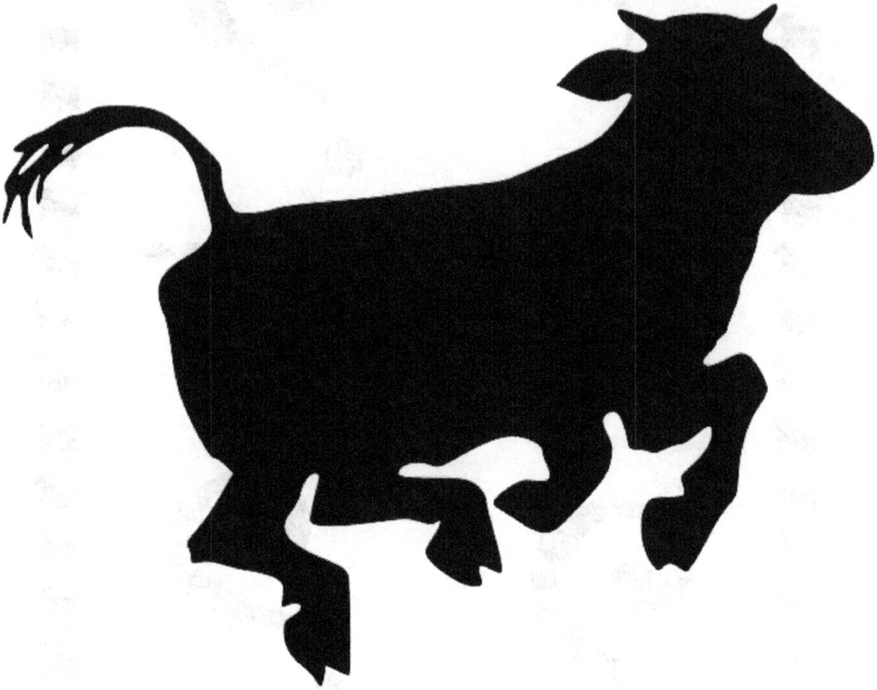

Chapter 1: Understanding the Carnivore Diet

You know, sometimes life has a funny way of nudging us toward something different when we least expect it. One day you're scrolling through your social media feed when you see a post about an all-meat diet. At first, you might chuckle, thinking, "How can anyone survive on just meat?" But then, curiosity kicks in. Could this really be the key to unlocking a healthier, more energetic you? That's how I felt when I first heard about the carnivore diet. I had just completed a treatment protocol with a functional nutritionist to balance my gut microbiome. She was convinced that the way to recapture my energy and health was through a ketogenic way of eating, *and* consuming at least twenty-five grams of fiber daily! Try as I might, I could *never* eat that much fiber. But my concern about carnivore was that it wouldn't feed my beneficial gut bugs, which I was told were now on their way to being newly-balanced. I needn't have worried; the carnivore diet has everything a human needs not only to survive, but thrive. It's not just another fad; it's rooted in human history and evolution[1]. So, let's kick off this chapter by diving into the fascinating world of our ancestors and their meat-centric ways.

The Ancestral Roots of Carnivory

Long before the days of fast food chains and supermarket aisles, our ancestors thrived on a meat-based diet. Evolutionary biologists and anthropologists have pieced together a picture of early human life where hunting wasn't just a survival tactic; it was a way of life. The evidence is fascinating. Our distant relatives, the ones who roamed the savannahs and braved the elements, developed physical adaptations that supported a diet rich in animal protein and fat. Our bodies were built for carnivory, from our teeth designed to tear and chew meat, to our shorter digestive tracts optimized for protein and fat absorption[2].

Archaeological evidence backs up this evolutionary narrative. Stable isotope analyses of ancient human remains reveal that our diet consisted mainly of ruminant animal protein. Imagine early humans sitting around a fire, enjoying a freshly hunted woolly mammoth. These scenes weren't rare; they were the norm. Animal protein provided not just energy but essential nutrients that were hard to come by in plant-based diets. This reliance on meat was crucial for survival and development[3]. The nutrient density of animal-sourced foods, such as vitamin B12, iron, and zinc, played a pivotal role in brain development and overall health[4].

The transition from a carnivorous lifestyle to agriculture marked a significant shift in human history, and not always for the better. The rise of agriculture brought about an increase in grain-based diets. While this shift allowed for population growth and the establishment of civilizations, it also introduced a host of health issues. Studies show that following the agricultural revolution, human health took a nosedive. We see a parallel rise in chronic diseases, including heart disease and diabetes, conditions that were virtually nonexistent among our hunter-gatherer ancestors. The decline in dental, bone, and general health post-agriculture is well-documented, with evidence suggesting that the reliance on grains has led to nutrient deficiencies and increased susceptibility to disease[5].

This brings us to the present day, where chronic diseases are rampant, and many of the top causes of death are linked to poor metabolic health[6]. Heart disease, cancer, and diabetes lead the pack, and they all share a common denominator: a high-carbohydrate lifestyle. Returning to an ancestral way of eating, one that prioritizes nutrient-dense animal protein and fat, is the key to reversing these trends. By embracing the dietary patterns of our ancestors, we can manage these modern health issues and perhaps prevent or even reverse them. It's not just about survival anymore; it's about thriving. And the carnivore diet offers a path to that vitality.

The historical reliance on meat wasn't just a matter of preference but of necessity. Our ancestors depended on animal protein for survival, and this dietary choice was mirrored by the development of animal husbandry in ancient societies. The domestication of animals provided a reliable source of nutrition and played a critical role in the advancement of civilizations. Through the ages, as societies shifted from nomadic hunting to settled farming, the role of meat remained vital, albeit diminished by the rise of agriculture. And the lessons of the past linger, urging us to rethink our relationship with food and the profound impact it has on our health.

Nutrient Completeness of a Meat-Only Diet

When you think about a diet consisting solely of meat, the first question that pops up is usually about nutrients. It's a common concern that a meat-only diet might fall short of essential vitamins and minerals. Yet, the reality is that meat packs a powerful nutritional punch. It's a powerhouse of essential nutrients like vitamin B12, iron, and zinc, which are harder to find in plant-based diets. For example, vitamin B12, crucial for nerve function and red blood cell formation, is abundant in meat but almost absent in plants. Interestingly, meat contains a form of vitamin C that is often overlooked. In the context of a low-carb diet, where the competition for absorption isn't fierce, the small amounts of vitamin C present in meats can satisfy our needs[7]. This is a paradigm shift for many who have always associated vitamin C with oranges and other fruits.

Let's talk about fiber for a moment. We've been told for years that fiber is essential for digestion, but what if that's not true? Studies suggest that fiber might not be as crucial as we once thought. In fact, fiber can cause intestinal disturbances like gas and bloating. You might be surprised to learn that many people experience improved digestion when they cut out fibrous foods. This is where the carnivore diet shines. By eliminating fiber, some individuals find relief from digestive issues, including constipation, they thought they had to live with forever[8], [9].

Now, let's focus on protein's role in nutrient absorption. Proteins do more than just build muscle and bone. They help transport vitamins and minerals throughout the body, ensuring that we absorb the nutrients we consume[10]. This critical function underscores the nutrient efficiency of a meat-based diet. When you consume meat, you're not just getting protein. You're getting a delivery system for a range of essential nutrients that work in harmony. Imagine a well-coordinated team ensuring that every part of your body gets what it needs to function optimally.

While plant-based foods can offer some nutrients, they often come packaged with antinutrients like gluten, phytic acid, oxalates, and lectins. These compounds, developed by the plants to defend against predators, can interfere with nutrient absorption, making it harder for your body to access the minerals it needs. By focusing on animal-based foods, you sidestep these issues, allowing your body to efficiently use the nutrients it takes in. The carnivore diet simplifies nutrition by removing the barriers that can hinder nutrient absorption, offering a more straightforward path to health.

Expert opinions lend weight to these insights. Dr. Ken Berry, a well-known advocate for the carnivore diet, emphasizes the nutrient density of animal products. Dr. Anthony Chaffee points out that many supposed deficiencies on a carnivore diet are myths, as the body is more efficient at utilizing the nutrients from meat. These insights from recognized experts provide a strong foundation for understanding why a meat-only diet can be nutritionally complete.

We are often told that you need to eat your fruits and vegetables, that carbohydrates are an essential macronutrient. Not true. Remember, an "essential" element of a diet means we must consume it because our bodies cannot make it. As you will see in the next section, there is no such thing as an essential carbohydrate[11] for the vast majority of humans.

As you explore the carnivore diet, remember that it challenges conventional wisdom about nutrition. It invites you to consider a different perspective, one where meat is not just a source of protein but a comprehensive source of nourishment. By cutting through the misconceptions and focusing on the science, you can appreciate the value of a diet that aligns with our evolutionary past while providing for our modern needs.

Evidence-Based Insights: The Science of Carnivore

When we talk about the carnivore diet, it's important to ground our discussion in science, not just anecdotal or personal stories. This way, we can see the broader picture of how this diet might impact our health. While the research on the carnivore diet isn't as extensive as one might like, there are key studies that shed light on its potential benefits. These studies, often free from the influence of pharmaceutical funding, reveal fascinating insights into how a meat-centric diet can promote fat loss and enhance metabolic health. Unlike the standard high-carb diets that can lead to spikes and crashes in blood sugar, a carnivore diet *"...naturally stabilizes blood sugar levels due to its lack of carbohydrates. This stabilization helps prevent insulin spikes and crashes, leading to more consistent energy levels throughout the day...*[12] ~ Nutritionist Judy Cho.

Moreover, the process of ketosis plays a pivotal role here. When our bodies enter ketosis, they begin to burn fat, instead of carbohydrates, for fuel, leading to more consistent energy and improved mental clarity. This means you're not just burning fat, you're becoming fat-adapted, which allows the brain to use ketones as a primary energy source. This adaptation can lead to better cognitive function, as the brain runs more efficiently on ketones compared to glucose. And when glucose is needed, the body has an incredible ability to produce it through a process called gluconeogenesis[13]. This means that even on a strict carnivore diet, your body won't be deprived of the glucose it needs for certain functions.

Beyond metabolic adaptations, the health improvements associated with the carnivore diet are noteworthy. Participants in various studies have reported significant reductions in inflammatory markers[14], a promising sign given the role of inflammation in many chronic illnesses. Inflammation has been linked to a range of conditions, from heart disease to arthritis, so its reduction can have widespread benefits. Additionally, the diet appears to support better overall metabolic health, with many people experiencing less fat storage and more lean muscle mass. This isn't just aesthetics; it's about reducing the risk of diseases linked to obesity and poor metabolic health. Seven of the top ten cause of death are associated with poor metabolic health[15].

Despite these encouraging findings, let's address the limitations in current research. The carnivore diet hasn't been studied extensively in modern medicine, mostly due to a lack of financial incentive. Unlike studies that support pharmaceutical interventions, which are often well-funded (and well-orchestrated), research on whole-food diets like carnivore lacks the same backing. It's also worth pointing out that many physicians aren't trained in nutrition to the extent needed to fully appreciate the benefits of such diets. This lack of emphasis on nutrition in medical education means that dietary recommendations often default to conventional guidelines, which have been influenced by industries with vested interests, including the sugar industry and certain influential food corporations[16].

However, here is a real-life account of a very limited (in participants) but very controlled study. In the 1920s, Vilhjalmur Stefansson, an Arctic explorer, along with a collegue, decided to challenge what people thought about diet by living solely on meat for an entire year. This wasn't just a random experiment for him—about 10 years earlier, he had already spent five years among the Eskimos, eating nothing but fish and other animal-based foods. He thrived during that time and was perfectly healthy.

When he got back to the States, Stefansson faced a lot of skepticism from scientists and doctors who thought eating only meat would lead to scurvy, malnutrition, or even worse. To prove them wrong, he and a colleague signed up for a year-long study at Bellevue Hospital, where they ate nothing but meat under strict supervision—they actually lived at the hospital. The result? Both men stayed in great health, showing that an all-meat diet could work just fine. You can read Steffansson's first-hand account of living with Eskimos and the year-long study in a two-part article he wrote in 1935[17],[18].

This sparked a lot of debate back then and is still a point of interest today for those curious about the carnivore diet.

By examining the data we have and acknowledging the gaps, we can make more informed decisions about our health. The potential of the carnivore diet to improve metabolic health, reduce inflammation, and stabilize blood sugar levels is a promising area that deserves more attention.

While we wait for modern medicine to catch up, let's remember the major 'study' during the first 290,000 years of our 300,000-year homo-sapiens-human existence, with men, women, and children participating: our ancient human ancestors, prior to the establishment of agriculture about 10,000 years ago, ate a meat-centric diet.

Comparing Carnivore to Keto and Paleo: What Sets It Apart

If you're exploring dietary options, you've probably encountered the trio of carnivore, keto, and paleo diets. Each offers its own set of rules and benefits, and while they share some commonalities, the differences are what make each unique. The carnivore diet stands out with its simplicity and focus on zero carbs. You eliminate all plant-based foods, therefore almost all allergenic foods, diving head-first into a regimen consisting solely of meat and animal products. This approach is quite different from keto, where the goal is to achieve ketosis through a balance of high-fat and moderate-protein intake, supplemented by low-carb vegetables and fruits. Keto followers often enjoy avocados, nuts, and leafy greens, which are off-limits for those on the strict carnivore path.

Paleo, on the other hand, expands on inspiration from the diets of early humans, focusing on whole foods like meat, eggs, fish, and vegetables. It allows for fruits in moderation, and the occasional sweet potato, which makes it more lenient than the other two. While paleo avoids processed foods and grains, it doesn't eliminate carbs entirely, like strict carnivore does. This distinction in macronutrient compositions—zero carbs for carnivore, low carbs for keto, and moderate carbs for paleo—sets the stage for how each diet impacts your body and lifestyle.

When it comes to health claims, each diet brings something different to the table. The carnivore diet's zero-carb approach can lead to rapid fat loss and energy stabilization by reducing insulin spikes and crashes. Many people report increased mental clarity and a steady energy supply. Keto also offers fat loss benefits but focuses on metabolic flexibility, teaching your body to switch between burning carbs and fats efficiently. Paleo, with its emphasis on whole foods, tends to appeal to those looking for a more varied approach to nutrition, often leading to fat loss through better nutrient density and eliminating processed food intake.

Lifestyle adaptability varies as well. The carnivore diet, with its straightforward meal prep and focus on meat, can be easy for those who enjoy simplicity and routine. You don't have to count calories or carbs or worry about portion sizes, making it a fit for busy individuals who want to streamline their nutrition. Keto involves more meal planning due to its need for macronutrient balance, and it requires careful tracking to maintain ketosis. Paleo offers flexibility with its inclusion of a variety of foods, making it easier to adapt to social settings and family meals, but it can involve more cooking and preparation time to avoid processed ingredients, and one must make wise food choices to maintain metabolic health.

Ultimately, choosing between these diets boils down to your health goals and lifestyle preferences, each with its own personal strengths and drawbacks; understanding these can help you make an informed decision. Whether you seek the simplicity, and ultimate nutrition, of carnivore, the variety of keto, or the even greater variety of paleo, it's important to choose what aligns best with your needs and goals. Each of these diets focuses on whole foods, ditching processed foods, and eliminating grains. The journey to better health is personal, and finding the right path is key to sustainability.

WHY

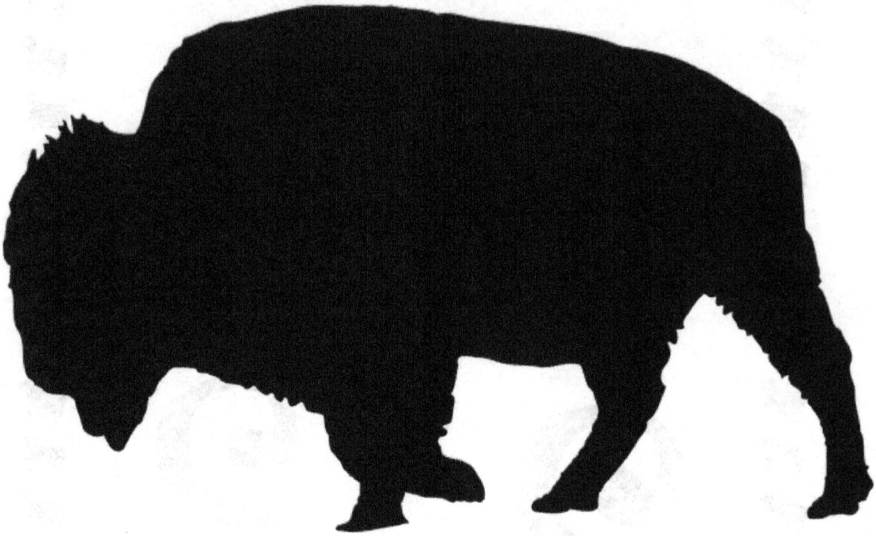

Chapter 2: Debunking Myths and Uncovering Truths About Carnivore Nutrition

Understanding Satiety: How Meat Satisfies Like No Other

Satiety is an intriguing aspect of the carnivore diet that often surprises newcomers. You might think of it as the feeling you get after finishing a hearty meal, but there's more to it than just a full stomach. When you consume meat, several physiological mechanisms kick into gear that help regulate your hunger hormones. Proteins, found abundantly in meat, play a crucial role in this process. They influence hormones like ghrelin, which signals hunger, peptide YY, and leptin, which signal to your brain that it's time to put the fork down. Ever noticed how a steak dinner leaves you feeling more satisfied than a pasta dish? That's the power of protein at work. Fats, too, are significant players. They enhance satiety by slowing down digestion, so you feel fuller for longer. This combination of protein and fat creates a one-two punch that keeps cravings at bay and hunger pangs from sneaking up on you.

When comparing the carnivore diet to plant-based diets, the difference in satiety is notable. Plant-based diets often involve foods high in carbohydrates and fiber, which typically don't provide the same lasting sense of fullness. You might find yourself reaching for snacks more frequently, as the quick-burning carbs leave you hungry sooner. In contrast, the carnivore diet's focus on high protein and fat leads to more stable blood sugar levels and prolonged satisfaction. Imagine eating a salad full of leafy greens and being hungry just an hour later; your body is calling out for nutrition. Now, picture a meal of grilled chicken thighs that keeps you satisfied for hours, until your next meal. The latter is a common experience for those following a meat-based diet, and it illustrates how effectively meat can manage hunger.

There's a significant benefit to this prolonged satiety—it can be a game-changer for body fat management. When you're not constantly battling hunger, it's easier to control food intake naturally. You might find that you eat less overall without even trying. The reduction in overeating tendencies is a direct result of actual nourishment and feeling genuinely full and satisfied after meals. This can lead to fat loss over time, as you're not tempted to consume extra food out of hunger or habit. It's a shift from the typical diet mentality, where calorie counting (aka starvation) is king, to a more intuitive approach where you eat until you're satisfied and then stop.

Beyond the physical aspects, satiety also has a profound psychological impact. Feeling satisfied after meals can reduce the likelihood of emotional eating. Many of us have turned to food in times of stress or boredom, but meat's ability to keep you full can help break that cycle. When your body's needs are met, the desire to eat out of emotion diminishes. It's a liberating feeling to know that your meals are meeting your nutritional needs, allowing you to focus on other aspects of life without the distraction of constant hunger or cravings. This balance between physical fullness and emotional satisfaction is one of the carnivore diet's unsung benefits.

Understanding these mechanisms highlights why many find the carnivore diet sustainable long-term. It's more than just the food on your plate; it's about achieving a state of balance where your body and mind are in sync, and that's a powerful place to be. The ability to listen to your body's natural hunger cues without interference from processed foods or sugars is an empowering experience. As you explore this lifestyle, you may find that satiety becomes a cornerstone of your well-being, helping you to cultivate a healthier relationship with food.

The Role of Metabolic Flexibility in Health Transformation

Metabolic flexibility might sound like a complicated term, but it simply refers to your body's ability to switch between utilizing carbohydrates and fats for energy, depending on what's available. Think of it as your metabolism's adaptability, much like a hybrid car that seamlessly shifts from gasoline to electric power. In the context of diet, this flexibility is crucial. It determines how efficiently your body can access and utilize different energy sources. Carb-heavy diets have left our bodies reliant on glucose, the sugar derived from carbs, as the primary energy source. This reliance can lead to energy crashes and cravings, and, if we eat carbohydrates at every meal every day, our bodies don't have the opportunity to tap into fat stores. The carnivore diet, with its focus on high-fat and protein intake, encourages a shift towards fat utilization, promoting a more flexible and resilient metabolism[19].

This metabolic efficiency offers several benefits, particularly when it comes to energy levels and mental clarity. When your body can effortlessly alternate between burning carbs and fats, you experience fewer energy dips. You may find yourself feeling more alert and focused, with the kind of sustained energy that gets you through both morning meetings and evening workouts. This is because fats, once tapped into, provide a steady and long-lasting energy source, unlike the quick spike and subsequent crash that often accompanies a carbohydrate-heavy meal, leaving you hungry again just a couple of hours later. Enhanced metabolic flexibility also means faster recovery times after physical activity, as your body can efficiently repair and replenish itself using fat as fuel.

Transitioning to a diet that promotes metabolic flexibility, like the carnivore diet, involves an adaptation period. During this time, your body undergoes significant changes as it learns to prioritize fats over carbs. You might experience what's commonly known as the "keto flu," especially if you try to rush the transition. This includes symptoms like fatigue or headaches as your metabolism recalibrates, and your gut microbiome adjusts. But these are temporary and generally subside as your body becomes more adept at fat-burning. Patience is key here, as the adaptation period can vary from person to person. You're retraining your body to run on a different kind of fuel, and once it clicks, the benefits become apparent.

Research supports the significant health impacts of enhanced metabolic flexibility. Studies highlight improvements in metabolic health markers, such as insulin sensitivity and fat oxidation rates. This means that your body becomes better at regulating blood sugar levels and burning fat, both of which are crucial for managing weight and reducing the risk of metabolic diseases. Moreover, a flexible metabolism is less prone to metabolic conditions like type 2 diabetes. By fostering metabolic flexibility, you're essentially gearing your body up for better health outcomes. This adaptability not only supports weight management but also overall well-being by minimizing the risks associated with metabolic disorders[20].

Addressing Nutrient Deficiency Concerns with Expert Insights

When it comes to understanding the nutritional power of animal foods, just how much they offer is eye-opening. Let's talk specifics. When you look at a juicy steak, you might see a meal, but it's so much more. It's a powerhouse of B vitamins, essential for energy production and brain function. Vitamin B12, in particular, stands out as a nutrient that supports nerve health and the creation of red blood cells, and guess what? It's a vitamin you won't find in plant-based foods. Then there's iron, crucial for carrying oxygen in our blood and preventing anemia. The heme iron in meats is more easily absorbed by our bodies compared to the non-heme iron in plants. Red meat also brings vitamin D to the table, a vitamin critical for bone health and immune function. And let's not leave out omega-3 fatty acids, especially abundant in fatty fish like mackerel, herring, salmon, and oysters, and less quantities in pasture-raised eggs and grass-fed meats. These good fats are known for their heart health benefits and their role in supporting brain health, linking back to the idea that nutrient density in animal foods can meet our body's needs in ways that are both natural and effective.

Now, you don't have to take my word for it. Experts in the field of nutrition, like Dr. Paul Mason and Dr Jennifer Geissert, have been vocal about the nutritional completeness of a meat-based diet. Dr. Mason has highlighted how the bioavailability of nutrients in animal foods often surpasses that of plant-based sources, meaning our bodies can more efficiently absorb and utilize these nutrients[21]. Dr Jennifer Geissert, a doctor of physical therapy and nutrition coach, echoes this sentiment, pointing out that animal foods provide a spectrum of nutrients that are difficult to replicate through plant matter alone[22]. Their expert insights underscore a growing recognition that the carnivore diet can indeed provide all the nutrients necessary for health and vitality.

But what if you're worried about missing something? That's where practical solutions come into play. Organ meats, like liver, are nature's multivitamin. They are dense in vitamins and minerals, including vitamin A, riboflavin, and folate, making them an excellent addition to ensure nutrient completeness. If you're not used to eating organ meats, start small. Incorporate them gradually into your diet. A little goes a long way, and they can be prepared to make them delicious and palatable. However, eating organ meats is optional; regular meat provides all the necessary nutrients.

Vitamin C: Absorption of Vitamin C competes with carbohydrates for transport throughout the body. When you eat zero, or very few carbs, just ten milligrams of Vitamin C is sufficient[23].

While nearly all nutrients can be adequately obtained from a carnivorous diet, there are certain situations where supplements might be beneficial. For example, if you're concerned about electrolytes[24], especially during the initial phase of the diet, an electrolyte supplement can help maintain balance and prevent symptoms like fatigue or cramps. Brands such as *NatureBell Electrolyte Powder* offer convenient solutions to keep your body hydrated and functioning optimally, using all-natural ingredients.

Another valid concern, which is even greater for someone who includes plants in the diet, is iodine. Thyroid tissue and breast tissue both need a good amount of iodine daily to be healthy. Farming soil has become increasingly devoid of iodine, and cruciferous plants complete for iodine absorption in the body, not to mention environmental competitors like bromide, chloride, and fluoride. As a result, everyone today needs to supplement with iodine for proper health, especially the health of the thyroid and breasts, according to Dr. Elizabeth Bright, and to the tune of about 12 mg per day (far more than the 150 mcg FDA recommendation)[25]. Dr. David Brownstein, another thyroid expert, starts most of his patients on 25 mg per day[26] (the link in this endnote has a fascinating interview with Dr. Brownstein, in which he talks about the woefully inadequate training doctors receive in medical school, and how he started with holistic medicine which healed his father of 20+ years of angina).

Ultimately, the key to addressing nutrient deficiency concerns is to understand the richness of what you're consuming and to listen to your body's signals. If you find yourself lacking in certain areas, especially in the beginning of your carnivore experience, explore ways to incorporate nutrient-rich organ meats or consider appropriate supplementation. And make sure you are consuming enough food; we women tend to shy away from food volume as 'fat loss by starvation' (can you say Weight Watchers…?) was ingrained in us from our youth. Eating enough quality meat and fat can truly satisfy without fat gain. By taking these steps, you can confidently embrace the carnivore diet, knowing that you're nourishing your body with foods that have sustained humans for millennia.

Dissecting Common Objections: Cholesterol, Heart Health, and More

Let's get right to it: cholesterol. It's a word that stirs up a lot of anxiety, thanks to decades of emphasis on numbers without a full understanding of what it really means for our health. Here's a simple truth: cholesterol is vital for our bodies[27]. It's not the villain it's often made out to be. Cholesterol plays key roles within your body, like building cell membranes, producing hormones, and even aiding in digestion[28]. Yet, many are caught up in the numbers game, worried about their LDL and HDL levels without understanding their functions. LDL (low-density lipoprotein), often labeled as "bad," and HDL (high-density lipoprotein), known as "good," are actually both essential. (NOTE: HDL and LDL are actually *NOT* cholesterol, but are transporters of cholesterol. These transporters, like high density lipoproteins, or low density lipoproteins, do the essential work of transporting cholesterol, the building block of all hormones among other things, to and from cells, ensuring that our body's needs are met. Yet you will constantly hear even doctors erroneously refer to them as cholesterol.)

Recent studies are beginning to shift the narrative, suggesting that cholesterol levels alone may not even be indicators of heart disease risk. It's a more complex picture, where the size and density of LDL particles might matter more than sheer quantity. Large, fluffy LDL particles seem less likely to cause trouble compared to smaller, denser ones. This means that a diet like carnivore, which can alter these particle sizes, may influence heart health in unexpected ways.

Now, let's address the elephant in the room: the fear of meat-induced diseases. It's a concern many share, driven by years of dietary guidelines that have painted red meat as the villain in our diets. As we explore the relationship between the carnivore diet and heart health, it's crucial to cut through the noise with evidence-based insights. Scientific evidence doesn't support these fears.

Remember that 290,000-year 'study'? And Vilhjalmur Stefansson, who lived with the Eskimos for five years eating nothing but fish? If eating only animal products was lethal, humans would have gone extinct millennia ago. That said, some modern studies have debunked the direct link between red meat consumption and heart disease, suggesting that other factors, like processed foods, industrial seed oils, and lifestyle choices, play bigger roles. It's crucial to differentiate between processed foods laden with additives and a diet based on whole, unprocessed animal products.

Let's dive into what the research says about heart health markers. For years, traditional 'heart-healthy' diets have emphasized reducing red meat consumption in favor of plant-based foods. They suggest that animal-based diets increase cardiovascular risk, but this isn't true, according to heart surgeon Dr. Philip Ovadia. It is dietary carbohydrates, not meat and fat, chiefly contributing to metabolic dysfunction and leading to seven of the top ten causes of death[29].

Let's talk about saturated fat, often the culprit in dietary debates. The idea that saturated fat contributes to heart disease is being questioned. Recent evidence suggests that saturated fat may not significantly impact heart health for most healthy adults. *"A few large and well-designed prospective cohort studies, which used validated questionnaires to assess diet and recorded endpoints in a systematic manner, were initiated recently. They demonstrated that replacement of fat with carbohydrate was not associated with lower risk of CHD* [coronary heart disease]*, and may even be associated with increased total mortality (29–31). Furthermore, a number of systematic reviews of cohort studies have shown no significant association between saturated fat intake and coronary artery disease or mortality, and some even suggested a lower risk of stroke with higher consumption of saturated fat..."*[30] This shifts the focus from demonizing saturated fat to understanding its essential role in diet.

Within the carnivore diet, there are protective elements that deserve attention. Omega-3 fatty acids, found abundantly in fatty fish, and in lesser quantities in meat and eggs, are celebrated for their heart-protective qualities. These essential fats help reduce inflammation and support cardiovascular health. The diet's emphasis on high-quality animal products means that you're likely consuming a decent amount of these heart-healthy fats. But it doesn't stop there. Meats themselves contain antioxidants, and when you're well-nourished, your body produces its own antioxidants. This combination contributes to an internal environment that supports heart health.

Concerns about red meat consumption often stem from misconceptions or erroneous outdated information. It's time to set the record straight. Red meat, particularly beef, is one of the most nutrient-dense foods available. It's packed with essential nutrients like vitamin B12—which you won't find in plants—iron, and zinc, crucial for overall health. The notion that red meat is inherently bad for you doesn't hold up when you consider the nutritional benefits it provides. The key is focusing on quality—choosing meat from grass-fed or pasture-raised sources (or the highest quality you can afford) ensures you're getting the best nutrition possible.

Journaling Prompt: Reflecting on Health Myths

Take a moment to reflect on your own perceptions of red meat and heart health. How have past dietary guidelines influenced your views? Consider writing down questions or concerns you have and exploring credible sources for answers. This exercise is about empowering yourself with knowledge and clarity.

As we challenge these misconceptions, remember that dietary choices are personal. The carnivore diet offers a new perspective, encouraging us to rethink traditional narratives and embrace a diet that aligns with our ancestral roots. Understanding the science and listening to our bodies can help us make informed decisions that support our health and well-being.

Cholesterol and Blood Lipids: Separating Fact from Fiction

Cholesterol almost always gets a bad rap, but it plays some pretty crucial roles in our bodies. It's like the unsung hero, working behind the scenes to support cellular structure and hormone production. Without cholesterol, our cells wouldn't have the sturdy membranes they need to function properly. Think of it as the foundation that keeps everything in place. Hormones like estrogen and testosterone, which regulate everything from mood to metabolism, rely heavily on cholesterol. And let's not forget vitamin D synthesis. The sunshine vitamin, as it's affectionately known, starts its life as cholesterol before sunlight works its magic, transforming it into the vitamin that strengthens our bones and boosts our immune system. Brain health, too, is intricately linked to cholesterol. Our brains are cholesterol-rich, and this lipid is vital for maintaining cognitive function and protecting against neurological diseases. So, while cholesterol might sound scary, it's actually a key player in keeping us healthy; without it, we would quickly die.

Now, let's tackle the myth that eating cholesterol directly jacks up your blood levels. It's a common misconception that what you eat directly translates into what's floating around in your bloodstream. The reality? It's not that simple. Several studies have shown that dietary cholesterol has minimal impact on the level of cholesterol in the blood for most people. Your body is pretty smart; it regulates its own cholesterol production based on dietary intake. On fact, about 80% of the cholesterol in your body at any given time, was produced by your body. If you eat more, your body makes less, and vice versa. Some research even suggests that people with higher LDL cholesterol—often labeled as the "bad" kind—might live longer, especially as they age[31]. The focus has shifted from just looking at LDL levels to considering the broader picture, including the ratio of triglycerides to HDL cholesterol, and other factors that paint a more accurate portrait of heart health[32].

What happens to your lipid profile when you embrace a carnivore diet? For many, the shift leads to fascinating changes. One of the most notable is the increase in the "good" HDL 'cholesterol.' Additionally, the carnivore diet can influence the size and density of LDL particles. Many carnivore followers experience a shift to larger, fluffier LDL particles, which seem less likely to contribute to plaque buildup, making LDL levels even less relevant when viewed in isolation.

Expert opinions on managing cholesterol provide some enlightening perspectives. Cardiologists and lipid specialists who are familiar with carnivore and keto diets often emphasize looking beyond traditional cholesterol measures. Dr. Ken Berry, a vocal advocate for low-carb lifestyles, argues that elevated LDL is not the end-all when it comes to heart disease risk. Instead, he suggests focusing on markers like triglyceride levels and HDL cholesterol for a more comprehensive understanding. His insights push us to rethink outdated paradigms and consider cholesterol's role within the broader context of metabolic health. This shift challenges us to scrutinize how we interpret cholesterol numbers, urging us to look at the whole picture rather than zeroing in on a single metric.

In the context of a carnivore diet, these insights encourage a more holistic view of health; understanding that cholesterol isn't the enemy it's often made out to be, and that the body is a complex system that thrives on balance. As we explore these ideas, remember to keep an open mind and consider how these revelations might influence your own health journey.

Understanding Inflammation: How Meat Can Heal

Inflammation, that sneaky culprit behind many chronic ailments, often flies under the radar until it forces us to take notice. It's a natural process by the body in response to injury or infection, but when it lingers, it can wreak havoc on our health. Here's where the carnivore diet steps in as a game-changer. Imagine a diet so streamlined it's like hitting the reset button for your body. By eliminating all potential irritants and sticking to nutrient-rich animal foods, you create an environment where inflammation struggles to thrive. It's the ultimate elimination diet. You've probably heard of C-reactive protein (CRP), a marker for inflammation in the body. Research indicates that a carnivore diet can lead to a reduction in CRP levels, which is promising news for anyone dealing with inflammatory issues. But the benefits don't stop there. For those with autoimmune conditions, the carnivore diet often brings relief. In fact, in a Harvard study involving 2,029 participants, a whopping 89% reported improvement in, or a resolution of, their autoimmune condition[33]. That's huge!

Now, let's talk about what makes meat such a powerful ally against inflammation. It's all about the nutrients packed within. Take conjugated linoleic acid (CLA), for instance. This naturally occurring fat found in beef and lamb has been shown to reduce inflammation. It's like having a built-in defense system with every bite you take. Then there are the anti-inflammatory amino acids, which are the building blocks of protein. Amino acids like glycine and taurine help modulate the immune response, reducing inflammation and supporting tissue repair. These compounds are abundant in meat, making it a potent anti-inflammatory choice.

Omega-3 fatty acids are another star player in the inflammation game. These essential fats, found in abundance in fatty fish like salmon, have long been praised for their anti-inflammatory properties. They work by reducing the production of inflammatory molecules in the body. While plant-based omega-3s exist, they come in a form (ALA, or alpha lipoic acid) that's less easily converted by the body to the active forms (EPA, or Eicosapentaenoic acid, and DHA, or docosahexaenoic acid) needed for these anti-inflammatory benefits. With meat, particularly fish, you get a direct supply of these beneficial fats, making it more efficient at combating inflammation.

So, when you think of the carnivore diet, envision more than just a plate of meat. See it as a powerful tool, equipped with the nutrients and properties needed to fight inflammation. The diet's simplicity and focus on whole, nutrient-dense foods allow the body to heal, free from the triggers and irritants that often accompany a more varied diet. By embracing this approach, you give your body the chance to thrive, unburdened by the chronic inflammation that has become all too common in modern life.

Gut Health Insights: Fiber Myths and Carnivore Truths

Let's start with fiber, often hailed as the champion of gut health. For decades, we've been force-fed the idea that fiber is key to keeping our digestive systems in top shape. But is it really the hero it's cracked up to be? Recent studies are beginning to question this long-standing belief, suggesting that fiber might not be as beneficial as we've been led to believe. Some research even indicates that a high-fiber diet might not significantly impact digestive health or disease prevention in the ways we once thought. It turns out that for many, reducing or even eliminating fiber can lead to improved digestion. The carnivore diet, by design, cuts out fiber entirely, yet many followers report a remarkable reduction in bloating and gas, leading to a more comfortable and efficient digestive process. It's time to reassess fiber and how it fits into our overall health narrative.

Switching gears, let's look at how this meat-centric diet influences gut bacteria. We know that the microbiome in the gut plays a vital role in our overall health, including our immune system, influencing everything from digestion to mood; there's a reason it is often referred to as the "second brain." On a carnivore diet, the diversity and composition of gut flora shift, potentially reducing microbes that don't belong and encouraging those that thrive on proteins and fats. This change might sound alarming, but it's not necessarily a bad thing. The gut adapts to the food it receives, and meat-based diets encourage the growth of bacteria that aid in breaking down proteins and fats efficiently. These adaptations may indeed foster a gut environment that aligns with our evolutionary nutritional needs, contradicting the notion that a diverse microbiome is inherently superior.

With fiber out of the picture, you might expect digestion to suffer, but surprisingly, many find that it's quite the opposite. Anecdotal reports abound of people experiencing smoother digestion without the bloating and discomfort often associated with high-fiber diets. When you eliminate fiber, you cut out a lot of the bulk that your digestive system has to work through. This can mean less strain and more effective digestion overall. For those who have struggled with digestive issues, the carnivore diet offers a new perspective on a healthy gut.

Let's not overlook the myths about fiber's role in disease prevention, particularly colorectal cancer. While it's true that fiber has been historically linked to lower cancer risks, recent studies are challenging these claims. Some research suggests that high fiber intake doesn't necessarily correlate with a decreased risk of colorectal cancer. This opens the door for alternative dietary approaches that focus on nutrient density rather than fiber content. The carnivore diet, with its focus on nutrient-rich animal foods, encourages us to look beyond traditional dietary advice and explore what truly supports our health.

Below is a simple chart, inspired by the informative article, *"Carnivore and the Gut Microbiome: Dispelling Myths About Fiber and Probiotics,"* on CarnivoreBar.com[34] This snapshot serves as a quick reference to reframe our thinking about fiber and gut health.

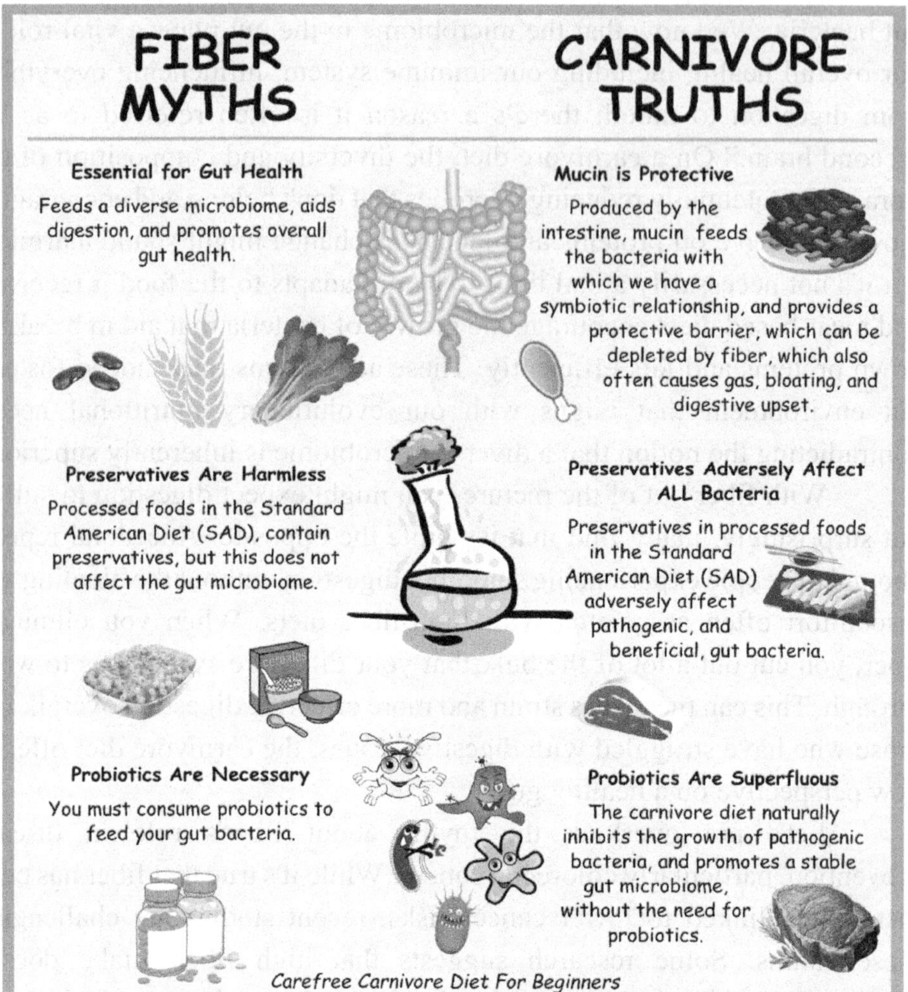

Stepping into the carnivore way of eating invites you to question long-held beliefs about diet and health. As you explore this approach, you'll find that the absence of fiber doesn't equate to poor gut health. Instead, it offers an opportunity to listen to your body and discover what truly works for you.

Exploring Mental Clarity and Mood Improvements

Imagine waking up each morning with a clear head, ready to tackle whatever the day throws at you. The carnivore diet might be your secret weapon for achieving this level of mental sharpness. At the heart of this clarity is using ketones as the primary fuel source for the brain. When you reduce carbohydrates significantly, your body shifts into ketosis, producing ketones from fat stores. These ketones provide a steady, reliable energy source for your brain, often described as a cleaner burn compared to glucose. This shift can lead to improvements in cognitive function, with many reporting increased focus, sharper memory, and reduced brain fog.

The anecdotal evidence of cognitive enhancements on a carnivore diet is compelling. People frequently mention a newfound ability to concentrate for extended periods, a valuable asset whether you're crunching numbers or chasing toddlers around. Scientific insights support these claims, suggesting that ketones may enhance brain function by providing a stable energy supply and reducing inflammation in the brain. This can lead to a more alert, attentive mind, free from the cloudiness or sluggishness that sometimes follows a carb-heavy meal. Users often describe the experience as akin to turning the dimmer switch up, where everything seems just a bit brighter and more vivid.

Beyond mental clarity, the carnivore diet appears to greatly impact mood and emotional well-being. Reducing foods that can cause inflammation and instability in mood swings is a key factor here. By focusing on nutrient-dense animal foods, the diet supports a more balanced emotional state. Users report significant reductions in anxiety and depression symptoms, which can be life-changing. There's something about the predictability and stability of the diet that seems to provide a sense of calm. Blood sugar no longer spikes and crashes, common with high-carb diets, which can lead to a more even-keeled disposition, allowing you to navigate life's challenges with a clear head and a steady hand.

As you consider these possibilities, it's worth noting that the path to mental clarity and improved mood is deeply personal. Exploring this path involves listening to your body and being open to adjusting as needed. The potential for a clearer mind and a more balanced mood might just be within reach, and the carnivore diet, with its bioavailable nutrition and absence of anti-nutrients, is the key to unlocking it for most people.

The Role of the Carnivore Diet in Managing Chronic Illness

When we think about chronic illnesses, conditions like diabetes, arthritis, and autoimmune disorders often come to mind. These are ailments that affect millions and can greatly dampen quality of life. One of the most promising aspects of the carnivore diet is its impact on chronic disease markers. Many individuals report marked improvements in this area, which is crucial for managing, and even reversing, many chronic illnesses. For instance, by eliminating carbohydrates and focusing on proteins and fats, blood sugar levels are naturally reduced and stabilized. Blood glucose, and therefore insulin, are no longer chronically elevated, a key factor in the management of type 1 and type 2 diabetes, and reversal of type 2. Additionally, those who adopt a carnivore lifestyle often see reductions in inflammatory markers, which are pivotal in the management of chronic diseases. When inflammation is reduced, the body can focus on healing and maintaining balance, providing relief from chronic symptoms.

SIDE NOTE:

"Insulin Resistance" is a misnomer. When carbohydrates are consumed, insulin is produced to carry the resulting glucose to cells for fuel. When a cell is already replete with fuel, in the form of glucose or fat, it "locks the door," not allowing the insulin to deliver the glucose cargo;

the cells are "resistant" to the insulin. When glucose is not allowed entry, it is instead stored in fat cells[35, 36].

Autoimmune conditions, notorious for their unpredictability and severity, may also see improvement with this diet. The carnivore approach strips away potential food triggers, allowing the immune system to recalibrate. Case studies abound of individuals experiencing remissions or at least a significant reduction in symptoms. For example, people with rheumatoid arthritis may find their joint pain and stiffness easing, allowing for more mobility and less reliance on medication. This isn't just anecdotal; healthcare professionals are noticing these patterns, too. Experts in diet-related therapies highlight the potential of meat-based diets in calming autoimmune responses. They emphasize that by removing common allergens and focusing on nutrient-dense foods, the immune system has a chance to reset, reducing attacks on the body's own tissues.

When it comes to cancer, there's a fascinating discussion around the role of glucose in cancer. According to Dr. Thomas Seyfried of Boston College, cancer cells are known to thrive on only glucose and glutamine. Cancer cells do not utilize oxygen like healthy cells do, but depend on the fermentation of glucose and glutamine. By removing glucose as a fuel source through a carnivore diet, and using mild non-toxic drug intervention to reduce glutamine when necessary, the cancer cells are essentially starved[37], making them more vulnerable to treatment. This makes tumors more operable, and reduces, or even eliminates, the need for aggressive treatments like radiation and chemotherapy. This research suggests that by depriving cancer cells of their fuel, you can effectively weaken them, offering a novel approach to cancer management. This concept, while still emerging, underscores the potential of diet as a powerful force against chronic illnesses. Next, Chapter 3 will highlight some amazing stories of real people being given hope through the carnivore diet.

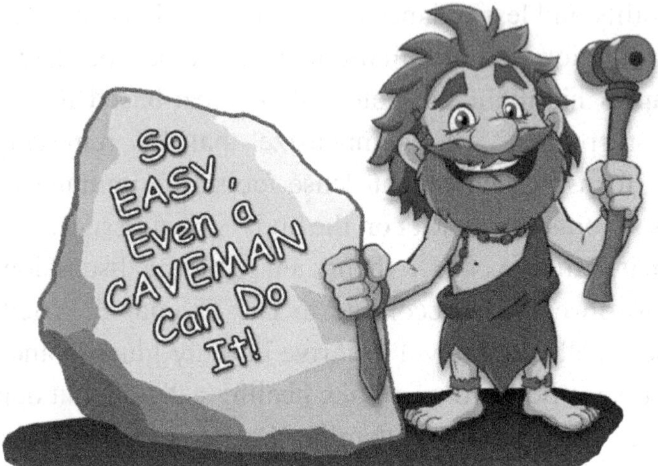
So
EASY,
Even a
CAVEMAN
Can Do
It!

Chapter 3: Success Stories: Real-Life Transformations

Below are stories of real people whose lives were positively and radically changed through the carnivore diet. Scan the QR code or visit the links below to listen for yourself.

Mikhaila Petersen Fuller was diagnosed with a plethora of conditions in her young life, and reversed them all: juvenile rheumatoid arthritis, juvenile idiopathic arthritis, major depressive disorder, bipolar, ocd, chronic fatigue, idiopathic hypersomnia, rashes, acne, chronic bronchitis, asthma, insomnia, PTSD, night sweats, freezing all the time, muscle weakness, nerve pain, fibromyalgia, IBS, histamine intolerance, SIBO, multiple chemical sensitivity, environmental allergies, food sensitivities, food allergies, numb legs, and red eyes. Her story is nothing short of amazing.

https://liondiet.com/my-story/

SCAN ME

Jason improved esophageal cancer, which had metastasized throughout his body, after being told he had just 3-12 months to live. Telling his story 15 months after diagnosis, he has renewed hope.

https://youtu.be/ciClMZsfhqQ?si=7zu_3OACoF75MboO

SCAN ME

Rebecca put her 10-year-long battle with multiple sclerosis into remission after just one month on carnivore.

https://youtu.be/gX2gQ3Cb1ZY?si=bTbA2LL19kBkEhrd

SCAN ME

Terry reversed chronic congestive heart failure with the carnivore diet.

https://youtu.be/fSTpFUyok-4?si=xpN0gSxTSVfJnBr1

SCAN ME

David put his incurable, non-operable very-high-stage-4 blood cancer into remission, and is healing the damage caused by previous chemotherapies, with the carnivore diet.

https://youtu.be/-LK2yyPwgqU?si=lqRTVDIcIY-IbfTi

SCAN ME

Sylvia reversed rheumatoid arthritis with carnivore.
https://youtu.be/vlg7i84uJE8?si=P8lsDxw9PkT5rXNQ

SCAN ME

Rebekah reversed more than 30 diseases diagnosed from a young age, and defied doctors who said she wouldn't live past 30 years of age, with the carnivore diet.
https://youtu.be/dWDTWqDvaZs?si=75ieuWamZUetga2m

SCAN ME

Mimi Morgan reversed Parkinson's disease with the carnivore diet.
https://youtu.be/Ty5l5ZF10qY?si=yOzxIKH5rUfTqWyu

SCAN ME

Kelly, carnivore for 13 years, lost 120 pounds and reversed chronic disease.
https://www.youtube.com/watch?v=CZ-qwRGNgjo

SCAN ME

Jordan Peterson (Mikhaila Fuller Peterson's father) lost fifty-two pounds of fat in seven months, overcame many ailments, including anxiety, depression, chronic gum disease (which is correlated with coronary issues), psoriasis, peripheral uveitis, and gastric reflux disorder, with the carnivore diet.

https://youtu.be/12Sza90czz0?si=ow7z6-m0GfGhdlzw

SCAN ME

Anji overcame Lyme disease, eczema, anxiety, and addiction by eating the carnivore way.

https://youtu.be/gGTNuIyIndo?si=T5CkYBLVPjZNQ7l8

SCAN ME

Chris Spath reversed type II diabetes, flesh-eating disease, and insulin resistance, with carnivore.

https://youtu.be/t0AXL88cbjc?si=E9Lvsy7ov1zzZCIF

SCAN ME

Laura Spath lost 120 pounds of fat in less than one year, and cured an energy deficit, acne, and hair loss, with the carnivore diet.

https://youtu.be/geBg4A4A0mc?si=oG7GNr60Bxi6pzVM

SCAN ME

Amanda lost 100+ pounds of fat and overcame an eating disorder on the carnivore diet.

https://www.youtube.com/live/qMiU5z5UlR8?si=kFABhKOiGh65MTe2

SCAN ME

David overcame depression, anxiety, obesity, acne, and helped heal a serious injury, on the carnivore diet.

https://youtu.be/sFIAD3JVuEk?si=TgggixZW5wUSHHZE

SCAN ME

Sarah Stringer lost over 100 pounds of fat, the aches and pains experienced upon waking in the morning, and brain fog, and was able to reduce medication for hypothyroidism, high blood pressure, heart burn, and eliminated decades of anti-depressants—all on carnivore.

https://youtu.be/9JJnWuowQt8?si=vTwR44wEyprZgrxE

Valerie Anne Smith overcame having anorexia nervosa for over 40 years, other severe mental health challenges like schizoaffective disorder, depression, body dysmorphia, and a severely underweight status with the carnivore diet.

https://youtu.be/nZbuQzSGf00?si=lTHImJE1FeIVZbRP

Maggie, born in 1941, has been a carnivore for 65 years, and still works her cattle ranch.

https://youtu.be/mnWdsEzx8F0?si=EHRm1omy4Xi0UuBL

In embracing a carnivore diet, it's normal to question and seek clarity about cholesterol and heart health, moving beyond the fear and focusing on what's truly important: nourishing our bodies with real, unprocessed foods. By examining the evidence and listening to expert voices, we can form a more balanced view. This isn't merely about numbers or fear-mongering; it's about understanding the role of diet in our overall well-being. As we continue exploring the carnivore way, it's helpful to remember that our health is a complex interplay of factors. Diet is the most important piece of the puzzle because it lays the foundation of the way our bodily systems behave and interact. Remember, we eat to live, not the other way around. Let's keep an open mind and stay curious.

Expert Opinions: Insights from Leading Health Professionals

When it comes to the carnivore diet, hearing from those who've studied nutrition and health can be incredibly illuminating. Experts like Dr. Ken Berry, and Dr. Paul Mason, who have championed low-carb and carnivore lifestyles, offer insights that challenge conventional dietary wisdom. Dr. Berry, a family physician who years ago was confronted with the fact that he himself was obese and ill-equipped to properly advise his patients, educated himself on human nutrition. He frequently discusses how modern diets, saturated with processed foods, contribute to a slew of health issues, emphasizing that a meat-based diet can be a return to nutritional sanity. Meanwhile, Dr. Paul Mason, who also became educated in human nutrition to overcome his own metabolic issues, dives into the nutrient density of meat, arguing that it provides everything our bodies need without the antinutrients found in plants. Their perspectives, grounded in clinical experience and research, provide a compelling case for rethinking what modern dieticians consider a healthy diet.

Yet, in the world of nutrition, opinions can vary dramatically. Just a little digging can reveal biases. Some critics of the carnivore diet lean on studies funded by big-food and big-pharma industries, which often emphasize the benefits of plant-based diets. These studies tend to highlight risks associated with high meat consumption, citing increased cardiovascular risks and other health concerns. But it's crucial to scrutinize the origins and motivations behind such studies, and the way in which those studies were conducted. Many healthcare professionals were educated in systems heavily influenced by pharmaceutical and food industry interests. In fact, about 67% of the funding for medical schools is supplied by drug companies[38]. Remember the adage, "He who pays the piper calls the tune"? This relationship can perpetuate certain dietary recommendations without considering alternative perspectives, or even the big picture. And the big picture includes the fact that drug companies do not want us to be well. They don't want us dead, either. They want us just sick enough to remain good customers. This doesn't mean all plant-based advice is flawed, but it does suggest the importance of evaluating the full landscape of research.

Doctors specializing in dietary therapies, such as Dr. Eric Westman of the Duke Outpatient Clinic in Durham[39], North Carolina, and Dr. Bret Scher[40], a cardiologist in San Diego, California, advocate for the use of food as a tool for managing disease. They point out that the body, when given the right fuel, has an incredible capacity to heal and maintain health, often without the use of drugs. These professionals are well-versed in both traditional and alternative approaches and recognize the power of a diet that aligns with our evolutionary history. They argue that returning to a more primal way of eating can unlock the body's innate healing abilities, providing a path to better health that's both accessible and sustainable.

Cardiologists and nutrition experts who advocate for low-carb and carnivore diets often emphasize the broader picture of heart health. Dr. Ken Berry highlights the importance of considering metabolic issues when evaluating heart disease risk, rather than zeroing in on cholesterol[41]. Dr. Paul Mason has discussed the limitation of medical education, such as teaching medical students how to write prescriptions and increase the dosages, but failing to teach them how to reduce and wean the patient from those medications when dietary interventions make them no longer necessary[42]. These insights encourage a more nuanced understanding of how diet impacts our health. In embracing a carnivore diet, it's normal to question and seek clarity about cholesterol and heart health, and finding, at the very least, a physician who is open-minded. Dr. Kiltz has put together a valuable resource to help us find just that[43].

It is important to move beyond the fear and focus on what's truly important: nourishing our bodies with real, unprocessed foods. By examining the evidence and listening to expert voices, we can form a more balanced view. This isn't merely about numbers, but understanding the role of diet in our overall well-being. As we continue exploring the carnivore way, it's helpful to remember that our health is a complex interplay of factors, and diet is the most important piece of the puzzle. Let's keep an open mind and stay curious.

As this section draws to a close, we've navigated through a spectrum of insights, from the tangible health transformations experienced by many to the expert opinions that lend credibility to the carnivore diet. This chapter serves as a reminder that dietary choices are deeply personal, and as varied as the individual reasons for exploring the carnivore diet. As we move forward, let's keep these insights in mind, ready to explore the practical applications and real-world strategies that will guide us in Chapter 4.

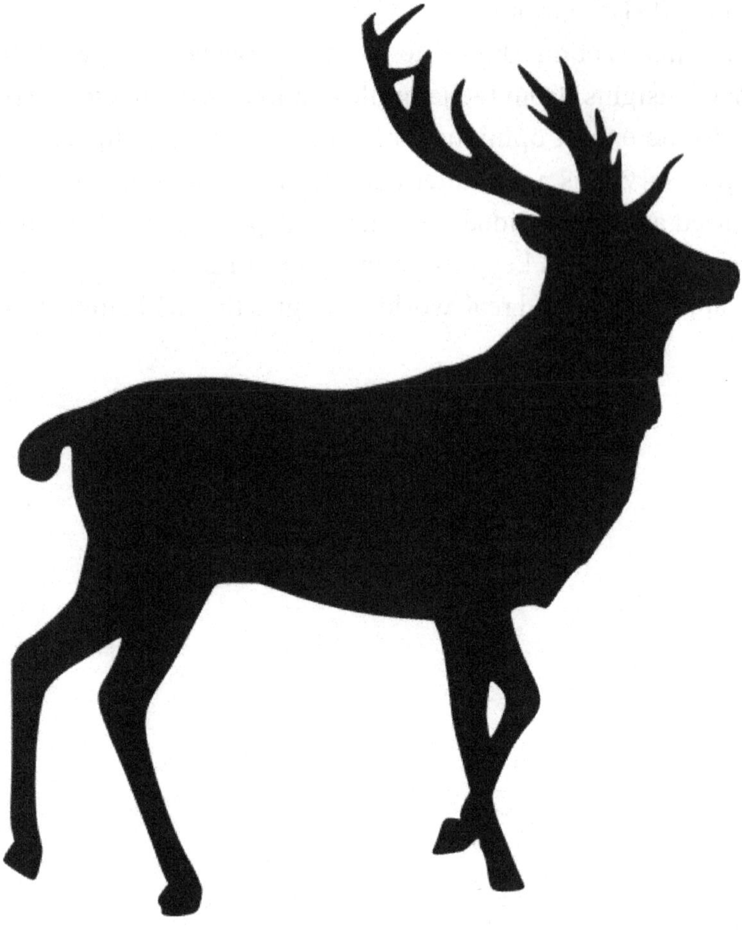

HOW

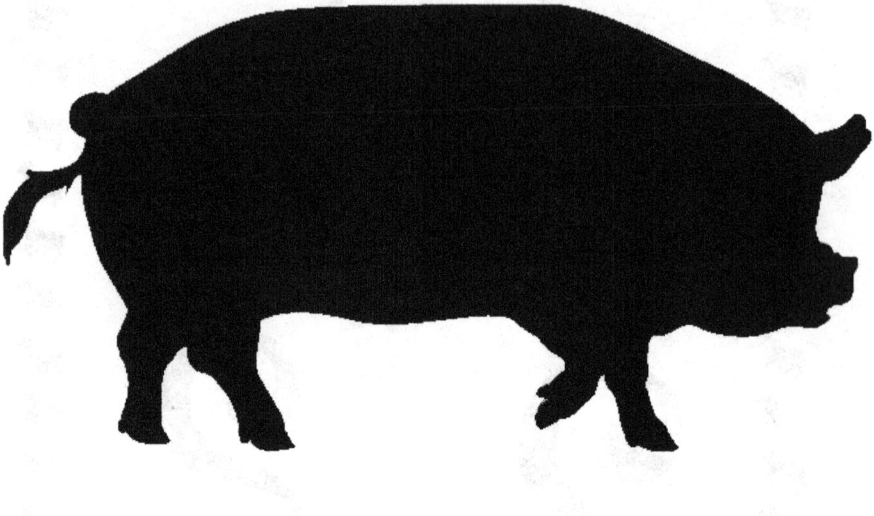

Chapter 4: Your Carnivore Journey: From Pantry to Prep

You're about to embark on a new path—a path that promises not just physical transformation but also a renewed sense of vitality. As you stand at this crossroads, setting realistic goals is your compass. It's easy to get swept up in the excitement of starting something new, but having clear, attainable goals can guide you smoothly through the first 30 days. Think of goals not just as an end point but as a roadmap, helping you navigate the ups and downs with confidence.

NOTE: If you are taking any medications be sure to let your doctor know that you have chosen to eat a very low carbohydrate diet, and that you would like for him/her to work with you to monitor your medication(s) and adjust as needed as you progress on your carnivore journey. This may require additional or more frequent testing. If your doctor balks, find another doctor who is more open-minded and willing to learn; the Dr. Kiltz resource (endnote 43) may help. A doctor familiar with the benefits of a carnivore diet will most likely also have knowledge of how one's bloodwork may change, what's important, and what isn't.

Setting Realistic Goals: What to Expect in the First 30 Days

The first month on the carnivore diet can feel like a whirlwind. Your body's adjusting, and you might notice some changes. Weight fluctuations are common as your metabolism shifts gears. You might drop a few pounds quickly, a mix of water weight and fat loss. Energy levels might dance to a different tune as well. Some days, you'll feel like you could conquer the world. Other days, you might feel a bit sluggish as your body adapts to burning fat for fuel. It's a natural process, and knowing what to expect can make it easier to embrace these changes.

There's also a psychological shift when you transition to a carnivore lifestyle, moving from a mindset of variety to one of simplicity. Instead of endless meal planning and calorie-counting or carb-counting, you focus on nourishing your body with quality meats and fats. It's liberating. You'll find that meals become less about ticking off boxes and more about enjoying what truly fuels you. This shift can be refreshing, giving you the mental space to focus on other aspects of life.

Tracking your progress is completely optional, but it helps many people to stay on course. Consider keeping a journal where you note not only the physical changes but also your emotional and mental shifts. Write about how you feel after meals or energy level fluctuations throughout the day. Some people find that apps make tracking easier, offering insights into their eating patterns and health metrics. But remember, it's optional. Do what feels right for you. The goal is to gather information that helps you understand your journey better.

Progress Journaling Prompt

Take a moment to jot down your thoughts. What are your top three goals for the first 30 days? How do you feel about this transition? Write freely, capturing your hopes and any apprehensions you might have. This exercise isn't just about documenting the journey; it's a tool to reflect and adjust as needed.

As you step into this new chapter, remember that setting realistic goals is about more than just hitting a number on the scale. It's about embracing a healthier lifestyle that fits into your life seamlessly. The first 30 days are just the beginning. With clear goals and a little patience, you'll find your rhythm and start seeing the benefits unfold.

NOTE:

"The gallbladder stores bile, which is necessary to break down dietary fat so that your body can use it for nutrition. When you eat a low-fat diet, the bile just sits there, becoming sludge and then stones. And the gallbladder becomes weak from lack of exercise[44]."~Effortless Menopause For The Savvy Woman by Marsha Shepherd Whitt. So, if you are transitioning from a low-fat diet, your gallbladder (if you still have one) may need a little help adjusting to the increased fat content of the carnivore diet. Drinking a tablespoon of apple cider vinegar in water just before and during a meal can help to release the bile needed for fat digestion. If you no longer have a gallbladder, apple cider vinegar is still very helpful. If you find you need additional digestion help, especially in the beginning of carnivore, a supplement such as "Gallbladder Formula" from Berg Nutritionals is a good product; I have used it myself.

Pantry Makeover: Stocking Up on Carnivore Essentials

Transforming your pantry to support a carnivore lifestyle is both an exciting and strategic process. It's about filling your shelves with the staples that will fuel your new way of eating. But before that can happen, you'll want to empty your pantry of foods that do not support your journey to good health. The first to go are obvious junk 'foods' like cakes, cookies, and candies. And don't give in to the begging of other family members to keep these around; they provide absolutely no nutritional value to anyone, but advance them down the path of developing seven of the top ten causes of death. If you follow my recommended transition schedule (below, in "Navigating Initial Adaptation Challenges"), you can clear your pantry of each type of leftover food items at the end of each week during your transition. Now, on to refilling your pantry with the essential elements of healthy eating.

Let's start with the basics: grass-fed beef, wild-caught fish, and animal fats. These are the cornerstones of your diet, providing the rich nutrients and healthy fats your body will thrive on. Grass-fed beef is preferred for its higher omega-3 fatty acid content and antioxidants like vitamin E, which are often lower in grain-fed varieties. Wild-caught fish, like herring, mackerel, salmon, sardines, and anchovies, pack a punch of essential omega-3s and are perfect for diversifying your protein sources. Then there's animal fats—think tallow, lard, and butter—which are not only delicious but also help you feel satisfied longer. Don't forget to save that liquid gold—bacon grease!—to drizzle over dishes for a smoky, savory kick. Strain it and keep it in a jar on the counter or in the refrigerator. Bone broth and organ meats, though optional, are nutrient powerhouses, loaded with vitamins and minerals that can enhance your diet's nutritional profile.

Quality is key when choosing these items. This means less inflammation and more heart-healthy fats for you. High-quality grass-fed meats are often richer in nutrients and don't contain the antibiotics and hormones commonly found in conventionally raised livestock. This not only supports your health but also aligns with the ethical and environmental considerations many health-conscious individuals value. When you invest in quality, you're investing in your health.

BUDGET NOTE:

Even conventionally-raised, grain-fed meats are far superior nutritionally and metabolically to the standard American diet. If your budget doesn't allow for premium options, rest assured that regular supermarket meats will still support your health and healing journey.

"Anyone can do carnivore, even those on a strict budget," Dr. Ken Berry puts your mind at ease:

https://youtube.com/shorts/EiIXZRwC1gY?si=Ap3oOkDkSmVQ8MEi

SCAN ME

Shopping smart is another piece of the puzzle. Locating specialty butchers and farmers' markets can make a world of difference. These places often offer fresher, potentially more sustainable options that align with the carnivore lifestyle. Plus, engaging with local producers gives you insights into where your food comes from, fostering a deeper connection to what you eat. To save money, consider buying in bulk. Larger cuts of meat or whole animals can be more economical, and you can always share the cost with a friend, and freeze what you can't use immediately. Buying in bulk not only reduces cost per pound but also ensures you always have a good stock of essentials on hand, preventing last-minute, potentially less healthy choices.

Quality fats are the backbone of a flavorful and nutritious carnivore diet, and incorporating a variety keeps your taste buds excited while supporting your health. Grass-fed beef tallow is a standout option, easily sourced on platforms like Amazon. It can even be rendered at home from raw fat bought at your local butcher shop. Pork lard and grass-fed butter bring their own rich flavors and nutritional benefits to the table, adding versatility to your cooking. Exploring these fats not only enhances your meals but also builds confidence in sourcing and preparing essential ingredients for your carnivore lifestyle.

Storing these essentials properly is crucial to maintaining their quality. Freezing techniques can greatly extend the life of your meats and fats. Vacuum sealing is an excellent method; it prevents freezer burn and keeps meats fresh for months; and it is ready to drop into the sous vide bath! If vacuum sealing isn't an option, tightly wrapping meats in butcher paper or freezer-safe bags works well. Labeling packages with dates helps you keep track of freshness and ensures you rotate your stock efficiently.

For daily use, having a small selection of meats in the refrigerator for easy access is ideal, while the bulk remains frozen until needed. This organization not only preserves quality but also streamlines meal preparation.

Investing time in your pantry makeover sets you up for success. With the right staples, you create a foundation that supports your dietary goals and makes sticking to the carnivore lifestyle easier. It's about creating an environment that aligns with your health aspirations, making your home a haven for well-being. Filling your pantry with these essentials isn't just a task; it's a commitment to a healthier, more vibrant you.

Meal Prep Mastery: Saving Time and Stress in the Kitchen

Let's face it, life gets busy. Between work, family, and all those unexpected little things, finding time to cook can feel like a juggling act. This is where meal prep shines. It's like having your own personal chef, ready and waiting in your fridge. By dedicating a chunk of time each week to prepare your meals, you reduce daily decision fatigue and make sticking to the carnivore lifestyle a breeze. Imagine opening your fridge and having everything you need right there, ready to go. No more last-minute scrambles or unhealthy takeout when you're too tired to cook. Meal prep puts you in control, saving time and stress throughout the week.

Let's break it down into a step-by-step guide to batch cooking. First, you'll want to start with pre-cooking proteins for the week. Choose a few different cuts—maybe some steaks, chicken thighs, and ground beef. Cook them all in one go. You can grill, bake, or even use an air fryer. Once cooked, portion them out into containers for easy grab-and-go meals. Think of casseroles as your best friend, especially if you're a busy parent or working professional. They're perfect for feeding a crowd or having leftovers for days.

When it comes to streamlining your cooking, time-saving kitchen tips become invaluable. Gadgets such as slow cookers and pressure cookers can be lifesavers, letting you cook large quantities with minimal effort. Just dump in your ingredients in the morning, and by dinner time, you have a delicious meal ready. Cleanup is a breeze too—one pot to wash and you're done. Speaking of quick cleanup techniques, line baking sheets with parchment paper or foil to minimize scrubbing. Keep a sink of soapy water ready as you cook to drop utensils and dishes in as you go. It saves time and keeps your workspace tidy.

Let's outline what a sample prep day might look like. Start your morning with a shopping trip to gather all your ingredients. Fresh meats, some cheeses, grass-fed butter, and any spices you enjoy. Once home, set aside the afternoon for cooking. It might seem like a lot, but once you get into the rhythm, you'll find it quite enjoyable. While the meats are cooking, you can prepare marinades or seasonings for variety. By the evening, you're portioning out meals and storing them. Use containers that stack neatly in the fridge or freezer, making the most of your space. Label each with the contents and date, so you always know what's on hand.

Sample Prep-Day Schedule

Morning:
8:00 AM: Grocery shopping for the week.
10:00 AM: Return home, organize ingredients.

Afternoon:
12:00 PM: Begin cooking proteins and casseroles.
2:00 PM: Finish cooking, start portioning meals.

Evening:
5:00 PM: Store meals in containers, label and stack in fridge/freezer.
6:00 PM: Quick kitchen cleanup, relax for the evening.

This routine not only simplifies your week but also helps you stay committed to the carnivore diet. It's about creating a system that supports you, making it easier to focus on what matters—your health and well-being. Meal prep isn't just a task; it's an investment in your time and health, making the carnivore lifestyle sustainable and enjoyable.

Navigating Initial Adaptation Challenges

As you transition to the carnivore diet, your body will undergo significant changes, and it's not uncommon to experience a few bumps along the way. Headaches, fatigue, and digestive shifts often accompany this transition. Think of it as your body recalibrating itself to a new, more efficient way of functioning. These symptoms, sometimes referred to as "keto flu," occur as your body stops relying on burning glucose (from carbs) to relying on fat as its primary fuel source. It's a bit like switching from regular gasoline to premium; your engine just needs some time to adjust.

To ease these symptoms, focus on a few key strategies. First, ramp up your electrolyte intake. Sodium, potassium, and magnesium are your new best friends. Consuming ample amounts of these can help mitigate headaches and muscle cramps. Incorporate bone broth into your diet or consider an electrolyte supplement (like *Naturebell Electrolyte Powder*) to help maintain balance. Staying hydrated is equally important. Drink plenty of water throughout the day to support your body's detoxification processes as it sheds excess glycogen and water weight. And don't underestimate the power of rest. Sufficient sleep allows the body to repair itself and adjust to the dietary changes with more ease.

Understanding the physiological changes your body is undergoing can lend some perspective. As you reduce carb intake, insulin levels drop, prompting your body to start burning stored fat for fuel. This shift in energy sourcing can initially lead to fatigue as your metabolism adapts. Your digestive system might also need time to adjust, particularly if it's used to processing a higher volume of fibrous foods or processed foods. This period of transition is temporary, and as your body adapts to utilizing fat for energy, you'll likely notice a resurgence in your overall vitality.

NOTE:

To make this transition smoother, consider a gradual transition over 4-6 weeks—this suggestion cannot be over-asserted. A gradual gives your microbiome time to adapt, reducing the risk of adverse effects like keto flu or skin rashes, or the inevitable war between the microbes. If microbes are deprived of their favorite foods overnight, they can begin to eat the mucosal lining of your intestinal wall![45], increasing the susceptibility to pathogens. Gradually transitioning from a SAD diet to carnivore creates a natural rise in beneficial bacteria that thrive on meat and fat, allowing them to gradually overtake the bacteria that rely on processed foods and fiber. It also gives your gallbladder a chance to ramp up production and ease into dealing with more dietary fat.

	SUGGESTED CARNIVORE TRANSITION SCHEDULE
Week #	**Eliminate through the week:**
1	Obvious junk foods like cakes, cookies, and candies
2	Grains like bread, crackers, pasta, and corn
3	High-carb vegetables and legumes, like potatoes and beans
4	High-carb fruits like bananas, and pineapple
5	Remaining vegetables
6	Remaining fruits

As foods are eliminated each week, increase your consumption of meat and fat. Pay attention to your satiety levels. If you're not hungry for your next meal, skip it. Eat when hungry, drink when thirsty. Listen to your body—when it needs fuel, it will tell you.

Expect any adverse adaptation symptoms to subside gradually over 2-3 weeks. During this time, your body is fine-tuning its metabolic processes, becoming more efficient at burning fat and maintaining energy levels. As you progress through this period, you'll likely find your energy stabilizing, focus sharpening, and overall well-being improving. Remember, any initial discomfort is temporary, and the long-term benefits are well worth the effort.

Communicating Your Choices: Talking Carnivore with Friends and Family

Stepping into the carnivore lifestyle can be an invigorating change, but sharing this decision with friends and family might feel daunting. Effective communication is key to helping those around you understand your choices. When discussing your diet, start by sharing your personal health goals. Explain how the carnivore diet aligns with your desire to boost energy, lose fat, or address chronic health concerns. By framing the conversation around personal goals, you allow others to see the diet as a thoughtful decision rather than a passing fad. This approach not only clarifies your intentions but also opens the door to more meaningful discussions about health and well-being.

Skepticism is a natural reaction, especially when it comes to diets that challenge conventional norms. Be prepared for questions about health implications and sustainability. Addressing myths head-on can help dispel doubts. For instance, when faced with concerns about nutrient deficiencies, you might share how the carnivore diet provides essential vitamins and minerals through nutrient-dense foods like beef and fatty fish. It's also helpful to explain how the diet can support metabolic health and potentially reduce inflammation[46]. Transparency, combined with evidence-based information, can turn skepticism into curiosity, support, and perhaps even a buddy to participate in the journey alongside you.

To foster educational conversations, consider sharing resources and information that have informed your own journey. Directing friends and family to scientific studies or expert opinions can provide them with a broader perspective. For example, you might recommend a seven-minute video from Dr. Ken Berry, which outlines the health benefits of a meat-based diet[47], or even lend them this book. Sharing credible sources not only supports your case but also encourages others to explore the topic with an open mind. This exchange of information can be a two-way street, where both parties learn and grow in their understanding of health and nutrition.

Building a supportive network is crucial for long-term success. Inviting your friends and family to participate in meal preparation or planning can be an excellent way to foster understanding. Host a dinner where you prepare carnivore-friendly dishes, showcasing the variety and flavors this diet can offer. This hands-on experience can dispel myths and demonstrate the practicality of the carnivore lifestyle. Additionally, involving loved ones in your dietary choices can strengthen relationships, as it emphasizes trust and mutual support. You might find that some are even inspired to join you in your health journey, creating new opportunities for shared growth and motivation.

Embracing Community Support: Finding Your Tribe

As you transition into the carnivore lifestyle, finding a supportive community can be a game-changer. It's not just about having people to chat with, but building a network that can offer both emotional encouragement and practical advice. When you're surrounded by folks who understand what you're going through, the journey is much more rewarding. They can help you navigate challenges, celebrate victories, and provide insight when you hit a roadblock. Knowing you're not alone can make all the difference, especially on days when motivation dips or questions arise. A community's shared experiences and collective wisdom can provide a solid foundation as you adapt to this new way of eating.

Finding your tribe isn't as daunting as it might seem. There are plenty of avenues to explore. Online forums dedicated to the carnivore diet are incredibly active and full of seasoned veterans and newcomers alike. These platforms are a wealth of information, offering everything from troubleshooting advice to meal inspiration. Social media groups, like those on Facebook and Reddit, are also bustling with activity. They provide a space for real-time interaction, where you can post questions and receive feedback almost instantly. If you're looking for face-to-face interaction, consider local meetups. Many cities have groups that gather regularly to share meals, discuss challenges, and learn from each other. These meetups can be a great way to form connections and establish a sense of belonging within the carnivore community.

The benefits of engaging with a community go beyond just having someone to talk to. They offer a platform for sharing experiences, which can be incredibly enlightening. By learning from others, you can avoid common pitfalls and discover new ways to enjoy the diet. Members often exchange recipes and tips, providing diverse ideas to keep your meals exciting and varied. This exchange of knowledge helps you remain motivated and inspired, especially when monotony threatens to creep in. Additionally, hearing others' success stories can be hugely motivating, reinforcing the benefits of sticking with the lifestyle and encouraging you to keep pushing forward.

Active participation is key to getting the most out of your community experience. Don't be a passive observer; dive in and contribute. Share your progress updates, no matter how small. Celebrating even the tiniest victories can boost morale and inspire others who might be facing challenges as well. Posting your success stories can be particularly rewarding, not just for you but for those who are just starting out and looking for reassurance that the diet works. Offering advice or answering questions also helps solidify your understanding of the carnivore way and strengthens your resolve. By giving to the community, you enrich your experience and help create a supportive environment for everyone involved.

Overcoming Common Mistakes: Consistency and Commitment

As you settle into the carnivore diet, consistency becomes your best ally. Yet, it's easy to fall into common pitfalls that can derail your progress.

One frequent error is inconsistent meal planning. Without a plan, it's tempting to make impulsive food choices that stray from your dietary goals. Having a reliable meal plan anchors your day, ensuring you have the right foods on hand and reducing the likelihood of reaching for less favorable options. Another stumbling block is giving in to cravings, especially during those initial weeks. Cravings are natural, but succumbing to them can undermine the foundation you're building. Recognizing these pitfalls early on positions you to address them effectively.

Here are some optional ideas to maintain consistency. Consider setting reminders and goals. These can be simple, like a daily reminder on your smartphone to prepare your next meal or a weekly goal on your calendar to try a new recipe. Visual cues, like sticky notes on the fridge or calendar alerts, keep your intentions front and center. They help reinforce the habit, making it easier to stay on track. Another powerful tool is keeping a food diary. Documenting what you eat holds you accountable and provides insight into patterns and triggers. It's a reflective practice that allows you to tweak your approach as needed, ensuring your actions align with your goals. But again, only if record-keeping is helpful for you.

Long-term commitment is where the magic happens. The benefits of the carnivore diet often reveal themselves over time, through gradual, sustainable changes. Perseverance means embracing these shifts and understanding that progress isn't always linear. Focusing on long-term health rather than short-term gains fosters a mindset that encourages patience and resilience. This perspective helps you stay committed, even when the going gets tough. Remember, it's about building a lifestyle, not chasing quick fixes. With this mindset, you'll find it easier to weather challenges and celebrate small victories along the way.

Motivation is a crucial component of consistency and commitment. Visualizing success can be a powerful motivator. Picture yourself reaching your health goals—feeling energized, shedding unwanted fat, or managing a chronic condition more effectively. Visualization makes these outcomes feel tangible and within reach. Rewarding milestones is another way to boost determination. When you reach a goal, whether it's sticking to the diet for a month or achieving a specific health marker, celebrate it. Rewards reinforce positive behavior and keep motivation high. They don't have to be extravagant; even small gestures, like treating yourself to a favorite activity or a new kitchen gadget, can be meaningful.

As you continue to navigate the carnivore lifestyle, remember that consistency and commitment are your guiding stars. They illuminate the path to better health and vitality, helping you overcome obstacles with confidence. By recognizing common mistakes and arming yourself with strategies to stay on track, you position yourself for success. The journey may have its challenges, but with a clear focus and determined heart, you're well-equipped to reap the benefits of the carnivore diet.

So, as you prepare to delve into the next chapter, keep these principles close. They'll serve you well as you explore the practical aspects of maintaining your health and nourishing your body. The path ahead is filled with opportunity, and your commitment to this lifestyle opens the door to a healthier, more vibrant you.

Tracking Progress: Measuring Success Beyond the Scale

When we think about tracking progress, the scale often comes to mind first. But let's face it, the numbers on a scale can be misleading. Your journey with the carnivore diet is about so much more than just weight. Let's shift focus to alternative success metrics that paint a fuller picture of your health and wellness. For starters, consider your energy levels. Are you finding yourself more vibrant and alert throughout the day? That's a win. Improved mood is another subtle yet powerful indicator. Feeling more positive and less stressed suggests your body is thriving on this nutritional shift. Physical performance benchmarks also matter. Whether you're lifting heavier or running longer without fatigue, these achievements show real progress. And don't underestimate the power of how your clothes fit. Sometimes, a loose waistband says more than any number on the scale ever could.

To make tracking these aspects easier, you might find it helpful to use a few tools—but only if you find them helpful; the object here is simplicity, not feeling overwhelmed. Journals are fantastic for documenting your meals, symptoms, and personal reflections. They offer a place to record daily experiences and note changes in energy, mood, or physical milestones. Apps designed for health monitoring can also be beneficial. They keep track of metrics like sleep quality, activity levels, and food intake, providing a comprehensive view of your progress. These digital companions can offer insights and trends you might miss otherwise, helping you make informed decisions about your diet and lifestyle adjustments. But remember, these tools are optional; the most important thing is to find what works for you.

Tracking self-reflection is a powerful practice that underscores the importance of tracking progress beyond the scale. Taking time for monthly check-ins allows you to see how far you've come and where you might need to adjust. Reflect on your dietary goals—are they still aligned with your needs and circumstances? Celebrate the victories, no matter how small, and acknowledge the challenges. This process isn't about perfection; it's about growth and learning. It’s a chance to connect with your journey on a deeper level, fostering a sense of achievement and motivation to continue. It’s about embracing the journey, knowing that each step brings you closer to the vibrant health you seek.

Remember the inspiration from hearing those success stories? These personal stories of transformation go beyond weight loss. They speak to the broader impacts on life—better relationships, increased productivity, and a newfound zest for activities once considered daunting. Sharing these stories can create a sense of community and reminds us that we are not alone on this path. It’s about celebrating the wins together, fostering a supportive environment where everyone can thrive.

Goals Journaling Prompt

Take a moment to reflect on your own progress. What non-scale victories have you experienced? How have your energy levels, mood, or physical performance changed since starting the carnivore diet? Jot down your thoughts, and consider setting new goals for the upcoming month. This reflection can be a powerful motivator, helping you stay focused and engaged with your health journey.

Self-reflection is a powerful practice that underscores the importance of tracking progress beyond the scale. Taking time for monthly check-ins allows you to see how far you've come and where you might need to adjust. Reflect on your dietary goals—are they still aligned with your needs and circumstances? Celebrate the victories, no matter how small, and acknowledge the challenges. This process isn't about perfection; it's about growth and learning. It’s a chance to connect with your journey on a deeper level, fostering a sense of achievement and motivation to continue.

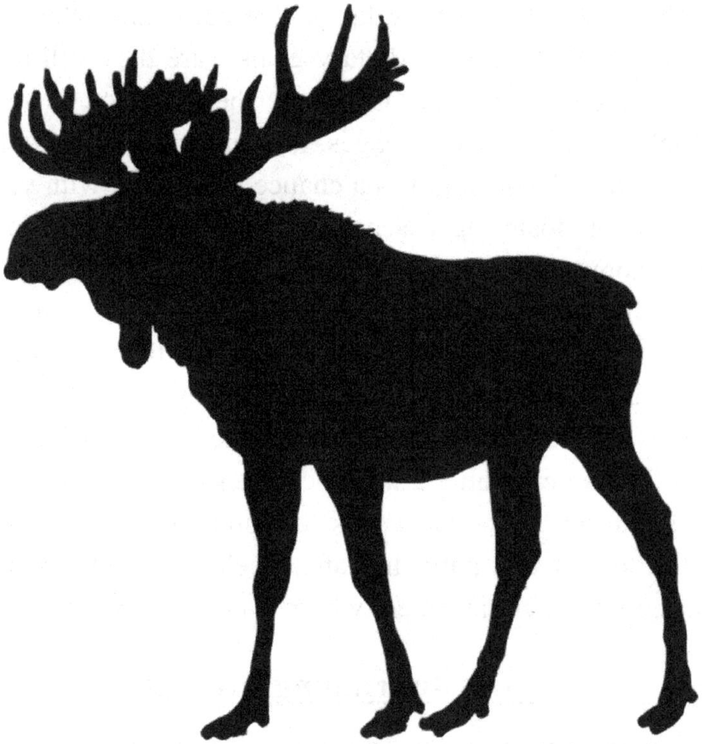

Chapter 5: 60 Days of Carnivore Meal Plans

Dive into 60 days of carnivore meal plans. These meal plans, and the recipes in the next chapter, are a goldmine of inspiration, showing how to mix and match common ingredients for satisfying meals without overcomplicating things. Most of the foods in our meal plans are pretty self-explanatory; most people know how to make eggs, and fry bacon or a burger. We have included recipes for some items that may not be so familiar to you. After that, there is access, through a dozen links and QR codes, to more than 50 additional recipes (no sign up or download required). Having no idea what to make for dinner is now a thing of the past. 😉

The meal plans below showcase the variety possible with simple ingredients and seasonings. They're flavorful, easy to prepare, and adaptable to suit your preferences! Feel free to substitute meats, or use another meat in place of organ meats mentioned, if desired. Some meats may need to be cooked in advance—this is where our handy Weekly Meal Planner can be very helpful (see Bonus section). Also, if you are doing strict carnivore, you may ignore any seasonings and sides mentioned.

We have provided meal plans for breakfast, lunch, and dinner. As you progress on your carnivore journey, you will probably find that not only are you not hungry between meals anymore, but you may not even be hungry for the next meal. Again, listen to your body; it will tell you what it needs. Eat when hungry, until pleasantly full, and drink when thirsty.

Much of the menu is straightforward, but some items might be unfamiliar to the average person. To make things easier, these items are marked with an asterisk (*) and recipes for them can be found following the meal plans.

Day 1

- **Breakfast:** Scrambled eggs cooked in grass-fed butter with crispy bacon on the side. Season with sea salt and a dash of smoked paprika.
- **Lunch:** Grilled chicken thighs seasoned with garlic powder, thyme, and sea salt. Serve with a drizzle of warm bacon grease.
- **Dinner:** Ribeye steak pan-seared in beef tallow, topped with a pat of herb butter (butter mixed with parsley and chives).

Day 2

- **Breakfast:** Omelet stuffed with shredded beef and cooked in pork lard. Sprinkle with black pepper and a pinch of oregano.
- **Lunch:** Pork belly bites baked until crispy, seasoned with salt and rosemary. Pair with a side of hard-boiled eggs.
- **Dinner:** Pan-fried salmon cooked in butter, garnished with a squeeze of lemon and fresh dill.

Day 3

- **Breakfast:** Ground beef patties seasoned with salt, pepper, and garlic powder, served with a sunny-side-up egg.
- **Lunch:** Roasted lamb chops seasoned with rosemary, thyme, and a hint of cumin, cooked in tallow.
- **Dinner:** Slow-cooked beef short ribs seasoned with salt and black pepper, cooked in bone broth with a splash of apple cider vinegar for depth.

Day 4

- **Breakfast:** Poached eggs topped with hollandaise sauce* made from butter and egg yolks.
- **Lunch:** Grilled pork chops seasoned with salt and pepper, drizzled with melted tallow.
- **Dinner:** Pan-seared duck breast with crispy skin, seasoned with thyme and garlic powder.

Day 5

- **Breakfast:** Ground pork sausage patties cooked in lard with a side of fried eggs.
- **Lunch:** Shrimp sautéed in butter with a sprinkle of paprika and lemon juice.
- **Dinner:** Slow-roasted beef brisket seasoned with salt and black pepper, served with bone broth on the side.

Day 6

- **Breakfast:** Soft-boiled eggs with a sprinkle of sea salt, served with bacon.
- **Lunch:** Pan-fried cod cooked in butter, garnished with parsley and lemon.
- **Dinner:** Grilled venison steak with a pat of garlic butter.

Day 7

- **Breakfast:** Pork belly strips baked until crispy, served with scrambled eggs.
- **Lunch:** Turkey drumsticks roasted with rosemary and garlic.
- **Dinner:** Ribeye steak cooked in beef tallow, served with a side of egg yolk dipping sauce*.

Day 8

- **Breakfast:** Omelet with shredded pork and a sprinkle of thyme.
- **Lunch:** Grilled salmon with dill butter and a squeeze of lemon.
- **Dinner:** Braised oxtail cooked with beef stock, salt, and bay leaves.

Day 9

- **Breakfast:** Bacon-wrapped eggs baked in the oven.
- **Lunch:** Seared scallops in butter with a hint of garlic.

- **Dinner:** Roast leg of lamb seasoned with rosemary, salt, and olive oil.

Day 10

- **Breakfast:** Scrambled eggs cooked in duck fat, topped with crumbled pork sausage.
- **Lunch:** Grilled veal cutlets seasoned with rosemary, sea salt, and a touch of lemon zest.
- **Dinner:** Braised oxtail cooked in beef broth with a pinch of black pepper and bay leaf.

Day 11

- **Breakfast:** Carnivore crepes* made with eggs and cream cheese, cooked in butter.
- **Lunch:** Seared scallops in garlic butter, served with a side of crispy chicken skin chips.
- **Dinner:** Pan-fried pork tenderloin medallions seasoned with sage and thyme, finished with a drizzle of bacon grease.

Day 12

- **Breakfast:** Fried duck eggs with a side of crispy beef bacon strips.
- **Lunch:** Slow-cooked beef brisket seasoned with garlic, onion powder, and smoked salt.
- **Dinner:** Grilled venison steak cooked in ghee, served with a pat of herb butter.

Day 13

- **Breakfast:** Sausage-stuffed portobello mushrooms* (for those okay with minimal plant-based seasonings).
- **Lunch:** Pan-seared liver (beef or chicken) topped with caramelized bacon bits.
- **Dinner:** Roast pork shoulder seasoned with fennel, garlic, and sea salt.

Day 14

- **Breakfast:** Omelet made with duck eggs, ground lamb, and melted gouda cheese.
- **Lunch:** Bison steak grilled with a touch of chili powder and smoked salt.
- **Dinner:** Grilled swordfish steak with a drizzle of lemon-infused butter.

Day 15

- **Breakfast:** Hard-boiled eggs sliced and drizzled with melted ghee, sprinkled with smoked sea salt.
- **Lunch:** Beef meatballs cooked in tallow, seasoned with garlic powder, oregano, and salt.
- **Dinner:** Slow-roasted lamb shoulder rubbed with rosemary and garlic.

Day 16

- **Breakfast:** Fried pork loin slices, seasoned with paprika and black pepper, served with scrambled eggs.
- **Lunch:** Crispy chicken thighs cooked in duck fat, garnished with a sprinkle of thyme.
- **Dinner:** Pan-seared trout topped with butter and a sprinkle of dill.

Day 17

- **Breakfast:** Bacon-wrapped egg bites baked in the oven.
- **Lunch:** Grilled burger patties (beef or bison) topped with a slice of gouda or cheddar.
- **Dinner:** Garlic butter shrimp sautéed with a dash of smoked paprika.

Day 18

- **Breakfast:** Carnivore pancakes* made with eggs and pork rinds, fried in lard.
- **Lunch:** Seared lamb chops with rosemary and garlic butter.
- **Dinner:** Oven-roasted duck breast seasoned with salt and thyme.

Day 19

- **Breakfast:** Chaffles* (cheese and egg waffles) with a side of bacon.
- **Lunch:** Beef ribs cooked in bone broth with a splash of apple cider vinegar for tenderizing.
- **Dinner:** Grilled pork steak seasoned with salt, garlic, and black pepper, served with a drizzle of bacon grease.

Day 20

- **Breakfast:** Soft scrambled eggs with cream, cooked in butter, served with a side of beef sausage.
- **Lunch:** Grilled salmon fillet topped with a pat of garlic herb butter.
- **Dinner:** Slow-cooked beef chuck roast braised in bone broth with a touch of salt and bay leaf.

Day 21

- **Breakfast:** Carnivore breakfast muffins* made with eggs, ground beef, and cheddar, baked in muffin tins.
- **Lunch:** Roasted pork belly slices, seasoned with smoked salt and cracked pepper.
- **Dinner:** Pan-seared duck breast with crispy skin, seasoned with thyme and sea salt.

Day 22

- **Breakfast:** Fried eggs cooked in tallow with a side of crispy lamb bacon.
- **Lunch:** Ground turkey patties seasoned with garlic, sage, and black pepper.
- **Dinner:** Grilled halibut topped with melted ghee and fresh dill.

Day 23

- **Breakfast:** Egg yolks whisked and cooked into a creamy custard, served with bacon bits.
- **Lunch:** Roasted chicken drumsticks basted with pork lard and sprinkled with garlic powder.
- **Dinner:** Venison stew* slow-cooked with beef broth, salt, and a pinch of smoked paprika.

Day 24

- **Breakfast:** Pork chops pan-fried in lard with a side of scrambled eggs.
- **Lunch:** Beef liver sautéed with onions (optional for non-purists) and seasoned with sea salt.
- **Dinner:** Grilled ribeye steak topped with a pat of truffle butter.

Day 25

- **Breakfast:** Poached eggs served over crispy pork belly slices, drizzled with melted ghee.
- **Lunch:** Grilled chicken wings tossed in butter and seasoned with garlic powder and paprika.
- **Dinner:** Pan-fried cod fillet cooked in beef tallow, topped with lemon butter and a sprinkle of dill.

Day 26

- **Breakfast:** Ground beef hash cooked with bacon bits and topped with a sunny-side-up egg.
- **Lunch:** Pork ribs roasted with a dry rub of salt, smoked paprika, and black pepper.
- **Dinner:** Slow-roasted leg of lamb seasoned with garlic, rosemary, and sea salt.

Day 27

- **Breakfast:** Cheesy egg bake made with eggs, cream, and shredded gouda, baked until golden.
- **Lunch:** Beef short ribs cooked in a pressure cooker with beef broth and a touch of garlic powder.
- **Dinner:** Grilled mackerel drizzled with melted ghee and seasoned with lemon zest.

Day 28

- **Breakfast:** Duck eggs scrambled with a splash of heavy cream and cooked in butter.
- **Lunch:** Crispy pork belly burnt ends cooked in their own fat and seasoned with salt and pepper.
- **Dinner:** Oven-roasted quail or Cornish hen brushed with butter and sprinkled with thyme.

Day 29

- **Breakfast:** Fried chicken liver served with bacon grease drizzle and a sprinkle of smoked salt.
- **Lunch:** Turkey drumstick roasted with an herb rub made of sage, thyme, and garlic powder.
- **Dinner:** Seared New York strip steak topped with garlic butter and a pinch of cracked pepper.

Day 30

- **Breakfast:** Bacon and egg cups (eggs baked in bacon-wrapped muffin tins).
- **Lunch:** Grilled lamb kebabs seasoned with cumin, salt, and black pepper.
- **Dinner:** Pan-seared halibut fillets topped with lemon and garlic butter.

Day 31

- **Breakfast:** Soft-boiled eggs with a side of smoked salmon and a sprinkle of dill.
- **Lunch:** Ground pork and beef mixture pan-fried into crispy meatballs, served with a side of homemade pork rinds.
- **Dinner:** Grilled venison steak with a side of bone marrow roasted in the oven.

Day 32

- **Breakfast:** Scrambled eggs with crispy bacon bits and a touch of heavy cream.
- **Lunch:** Beef tenderloin medallions grilled with rosemary and garlic butter.
- **Dinner:** Slow-cooked oxtail stew with beef broth, bay leaves, and salt.

Day 33

- **Breakfast:** Carnivore egg muffins made with eggs, sausage, and cheese, baked in muffin tins.
- **Lunch:** Pork chops pan-fried in ghee, sprinkled with smoked sea salt.
- **Dinner:** Grilled salmon with a lemon-butter sauce and fresh parsley.

Day 34

- **Breakfast:** Sausage and egg scramble cooked in beef tallow, topped with cheddar.
- **Lunch:** Beef brisket cooked low and slow with garlic, onion powder, and a touch of salt.
- **Dinner:** Pan-seared shrimp cooked in butter with a sprinkle of smoked paprika.

Day 35

- **Breakfast:** Scrambled eggs cooked in bacon grease with a side of crispy pork belly.
- **Lunch:** Grilled ribeye steak seasoned with garlic and rosemary, served with a dollop of herb butter.
- **Dinner:** Slow-cooked lamb stew with bone broth, rosemary, and salt.

Day 36

- **Breakfast:** Beef liver sautéed in butter with a sprinkle of salt, served with soft-boiled eggs.
- **Lunch:** Grilled bison burgers topped with melted cheese (optional) and served with a side of crispy chicken skin.
- **Dinner:** Roasted duck leg cooked in duck fat, seasoned with thyme and cracked pepper.

Day 37

- **Breakfast:** Carnivore egg bake made with eggs, ground sausage, and cheese, baked until golden.
- **Lunch:** Grilled pork belly with a side of creamy scrambled eggs cooked in butter.
- **Dinner:** Pan-seared trout fillets cooked in ghee, seasoned with a pinch of smoked paprika.

Day 38

- **Breakfast:** Duck eggs fried in pork lard, served with a side of grilled venison sausage.
- **Lunch:** Seared ribeye steak topped with a dollop of garlic butter and served with a side of crispy bacon.
- **Dinner:** Slow-braised beef shank cooked in beef broth with salt and bay leaves.

Day 39

- **Breakfast:** Fried eggs with a side of smoked salmon and a drizzle of melted ghee.
- **Lunch:** Ground beef cooked in beef tallow, seasoned with salt and garlic, served with crispy chicken wings.
- **Dinner:** Grilled swordfish steaks with a squeeze of lemon and a side of crispy pork rinds.

Day 40

- **Breakfast:** Egg and sausage muffins, baked with eggs, ground sausage, and cheese.
- **Lunch:** Grilled chicken thighs, brushed with ghee and seasoned with thyme and black pepper.
- **Dinner:** Pan-seared lamb chops cooked in tallow, seasoned with rosemary and garlic.

Day 41

- **Breakfast:** Soft scrambled eggs with crispy bacon bits and a sprinkle of smoked sea salt.
- **Lunch:** Grilled pork steaks seasoned with paprika and served with a side of bacon-wrapped asparagus (optional).
- **Dinner:** Beef stew made with short ribs, slow-cooked in bone broth and seasoned with bay leaves and thyme.

Day 42

- **Breakfast:** Carnivore pancakes made from eggs, pork rinds, and cream, cooked in lard.
- **Lunch:** Baked salmon fillets topped with a garlic butter sauce and a squeeze of lemon.
- **Dinner:** Grilled chicken breast, seasoned with a blend of rosemary, garlic, and sea salt.

Day 43

- **Breakfast:** Fried duck eggs served over a bed of crispy pork belly slices.
- **Lunch:** Ground bison meatballs cooked in beef tallow, seasoned with oregano and garlic powder.
- **Dinner:** Roasted prime rib with bone marrow butter* and a side of crispy chicken skin.

Day 44

- **Breakfast:** Scrambled eggs cooked in butter, served with a side of crispy sausage patties.
- **Lunch:** Grilled shrimp cooked in ghee and served with a side of bacon-wrapped beef tenderloin bites.
- **Dinner:** Pan-seared venison steaks, cooked in butter and seasoned with salt, pepper, and rosemary.

Day 45

- **Breakfast:** Poached eggs with a side of crispy turkey bacon.
- **Lunch:** Grilled beef heart slices, seasoned with salt and pepper, served with a side of pork rinds.
- **Dinner:** Pan-seared duck breast, cooked to perfection with crispy skin, topped with a bit of ghee and thyme.

Day 46

- **Breakfast:** Carnivore-style frittata made with eggs, ground beef, and cheddar, cooked until golden.
- **Lunch:** Grilled lamb kebabs marinated in olive oil, garlic, and rosemary.
- **Dinner:** Slow-cooked oxtail stew with beef broth and bay leaves, seasoned with salt and pepper.

Day 47

- **Breakfast:** Scrambled eggs with sausage links, cooked in beef tallow.
- **Lunch:** Pan-seared cod fillets, topped with a dollop of lemon butter and a sprinkle of fresh parsley.
- **Dinner:** Grilled bone-in ribeye steak, seasoned with salt and black pepper, served with a side of crispy bacon.

Day 48

- **Breakfast:** Fried eggs cooked in duck fat, served with a side of grilled venison sausage.
- **Lunch:** Pork belly slices, roasted until crispy, seasoned with sea salt and smoked paprika.
- **Dinner:** Grilled shrimp with garlic butter and a sprinkle of chili flakes, served with a side of crispy pork skin.

- **Breakfast:** Egg yolk custard* made with heavy cream, vanilla, and a touch of sea salt.
- **Lunch:** Ground beef cooked in beef tallow, seasoned with cumin and paprika, served with a side of crispy chicken wings.
- **Dinner:** Roasted chicken thighs, seasoned with garlic, thyme, and salt, served with a side of bone marrow roasted in the oven.

Day 50

- **Breakfast:** Scrambled eggs with ground pork and cheddar cheese, cooked in butter.
- **Lunch:** Grilled turkey burgers with melted gouda cheese, served with a side of crispy bacon.
- **Dinner:** Pan-seared scallops with a garlic-butter sauce and a sprinkle of fresh parsley.

Day 51

- **Breakfast:** Soft-boiled eggs with a side of smoked salmon and a drizzle of melted ghee.
- **Lunch:** Grilled beef heart steak, seasoned with salt, pepper, and garlic powder, served with crispy pork rinds.
- **Dinner:** Slow-roasted duck leg with rosemary, thyme, and a side of roasted chicken skin.

Day 52

- **Breakfast:** Carnivore omelet made with eggs, leftover grilled steak, and melted butter.
- **Lunch:** Grilled lamb chops, marinated in olive oil, garlic, and fresh mint.
- **Dinner:** Roasted pork belly with crispy crackling, served with a side of sautéed liver cooked in beef tallow.

Day 53

- **Breakfast:** Beef liver cooked in butter with scrambled eggs.
- **Lunch:** Pan-seared shrimp cooked in ghee, served with a side of beef jerky and pork cracklings.
- **Dinner:** Grilled salmon fillets with lemon-butter sauce and a side of crispy bacon.

Day 54

- **Breakfast:** Sausage patties with eggs cooked in duck fat, seasoned with a sprinkle of smoked salt.
- **Lunch:** Grilled pork tenderloin, rubbed with salt, pepper, and garlic powder, served with a side of crispy turkey bacon.
- **Dinner:** Pan-seared ribeye steak with a garlic-butter drizzle and a side of crispy chicken skin.

Day 55

- **Breakfast:** Scrambled eggs cooked in beef tallow, served with crispy pork belly.
- **Lunch:** Grilled venison steak, seasoned with salt, black pepper, and garlic powder, served with a side of bone marrow.
- **Dinner:** Slow-braised short ribs in beef broth with rosemary and thyme, served with roasted pork skin.

Day 56

- **Breakfast:** Soft-boiled eggs with a side of crispy bacon and grilled beef heart slices.
- **Lunch:** Grilled chicken thighs brushed with olive oil and lemon, served with a side of beef tallow-fried eggs.
- **Dinner:** Pan-seared swordfish steaks, cooked in ghee, seasoned with lemon and fresh thyme.

Day 57

- **Breakfast:** Beef liver cooked in butter, served with a side of scrambled eggs and pork sausage.
- **Lunch:** Grilled lamb chops, seasoned with garlic, rosemary, and salt, served with a side of crispy chicken skin.
- **Dinner:** Slow-roasted brisket cooked with salt and pepper, served with a side of bone marrow.

Day 58

- **Breakfast:** Carnivore egg muffins made with eggs, cheese, and ground pork, baked until golden.
- **Lunch:** Pan-seared shrimp in garlic butter, served with a side of crispy pork belly.
- **Dinner:** Grilled ribeye steak with a side of sautéed mushrooms cooked in beef tallow.

Day 59

- **Breakfast:** Duck eggs scrambled in ghee, served with grilled sausage patties.
- **Lunch:** Bison burgers topped with melted cheese (optional) and a side of pork rinds.
- **Dinner:** Pan-seared venison medallions, cooked in butter, and served with a side of crispy bacon.

Day 60

- **Breakfast:** Eggs scrambled with ground beef and melted cheddar cheese, cooked in butter.
- **Lunch:** Grilled chicken wings, seasoned with salt, pepper, and smoked paprika, served with a side of crispy pork cracklings.
- **Dinner:** Slow-cooked lamb shank with rosemary and garlic, served with a side of roasted bone marrow.

Below are recipes for items in our 60-day meal plan marked with an asterisk (*) that might need clarification.

Hollandaise Sauce (Butter & Eggs)

Ingredients:

- 4 large egg yolks
- 1 cup (2 sticks) unsalted butter, melted
- 1 tbsp fresh lemon juice
- Salt, to taste
- A pinch of cayenne pepper (optional)

Instructions:

1. In a heatproof bowl, whisk together the egg yolks and lemon juice until well combined.
2. Heat the bowl over a double boiler. Whisk constantly until the egg yolks are thickened and pale.
3. Slowly drizzle in the melted butter, a little at a time, while continuing to whisk. The sauce should thicken and become creamy.
4. Season with salt and cayenne pepper, and serve warm over eggs or steak.

Egg Yolk Dipping Sauce

Ingredients:

- 4 large egg yolks
- 1 tbsp apple cider vinegar
- 1 tsp Dijon mustard (optional)
- Salt, to taste
- A pinch of black pepper

Instructions:

1. In a small bowl, whisk together the egg yolks, vinegar, mustard (if using), salt, and pepper.
2. Whisk constantly until the mixture thickens slightly.
3. Serve as a dipping sauce with steak or vegetables.

Carnivore Crepes (Eggs & Cream Cheese)

Ingredients:

- 2 large eggs
- 2 oz cream cheese, softened
- 1 tbsp butter (for cooking)
- Pinch of salt

Instructions:

1. In a blender or bowl, blend the eggs, cream cheese, and salt until smooth.
2. Heat butter in a non-stick pan over medium heat.
3. Pour in a small amount of the mixture, swirling the pan to spread it thin.
4. Cook for 1-2 minutes per side, until golden and firm.
5. Serve with your choice of carnivore-friendly toppings (like bacon or ground beef).

Sausage-Stuffed Portobello Mushrooms

Ingredients:

- 4 large Portobello mushrooms, stems removed
- 1 lb ground sausage
- 1/2 cup shredded cheddar cheese
- Salt and pepper to taste
- Fresh herbs (optional)

Instructions:

1. Preheat oven to 375°F (190°C).
2. Remove the stems from the mushrooms and place them on a baking sheet.
3. Cook the sausage in a pan until browned, then drain excess fat.
4. Mix the cooked sausage with the cheese and season with salt and pepper.
5. Stuff the mushroom caps with the sausage mixture.
6. Bake for 15-20 minutes, until mushrooms are tender and cheese is melted.

Carnivore Pancakes (Eggs & Pork Rinds)

Ingredients:

- 3 large eggs
- 1 cup crushed pork rinds
- 1/4 tsp baking soda (optional)
- 1 tbsp butter for cooking
- Pinch of salt

Instructions:

1. Beat the eggs in a bowl, then stir in the crushed pork rinds and baking soda.
2. Heat butter in a skillet over medium heat.
3. Pour in small portions of the pancake mixture, cooking until bubbles form on the surface. Flip and cook until golden.
4. Serve with butter or sugar-free syrup.

Chaffles (Cheese & Egg Waffles)

Ingredients:

- 1 large egg
- 1/2 cup shredded cheese (cheddar or mozzarella)
- 1 tbsp almond flour (optional for texture)

- Salt, to taste

Instructions:

1. Preheat the waffle iron.
2. Whisk the egg in a bowl, then stir in the shredded cheese and almond flour (if using).
3. Pour the mixture into the waffle iron and cook until crispy and golden.
4. Serve as a breakfast or sandwich base.

Carnivore Breakfast Muffins (Eggs, Ground Beef & Cheddar)

Ingredients:

- 6 large eggs
- 1 lb ground beef
- 1/2 cup shredded cheddar cheese
- Salt and pepper, to taste
- 1/2 tsp garlic powder (optional)

Instructions:

1. Preheat oven to 375°F (190°C) and grease a muffin tin.
2. Brown the ground beef in a pan and season with salt, pepper, and garlic powder.
3. Whisk the eggs and cheese together in a bowl.
4. Add the cooked beef to the egg mixture and stir.
5. Pour into the muffin tin, filling each cup about 2/3 full.
6. Bake for 15-18 minutes, until muffins are set and golden.

   You may use to base recipe above and substitute a different meat or a combination of different meats, for varieties of muffins.

Venison Stew

Ingredients:

- 2 lbs venison stew meat
- 1 medium onion, chopped
- 3 cloves garlic, minced
- 4 cups beef broth
- 2 tbsp olive oil
- 1 tsp thyme
- Salt and pepper to taste

Instructions:

1. Heat olive oil in a large pot over medium heat. Brown the venison stew meat in batches.
2. Add the onion and garlic to the pot, cooking until softened.
3. Pour in the beef broth and bring to a simmer.
4. Stir in thyme, salt, and pepper.
5. Simmer for 1.5-2 hours, until venison is tender.

Bone Marrow Butter

Ingredients:

- 4 oz bone marrow (from beef bones)
- 1/2 cup unsalted butter, softened
- Salt, to taste
- Fresh parsley, finely chopped (optional)

Instructions:

1. Roast bone marrow in the oven at 400°F (200°C) for 20-30 minutes, until the marrow is soft and golden.
2. Scoop out the marrow and mix with softened butter.
3. Stir in salt to taste, and fresh parsley if desired.
4. Serve over steaks or roasted meats.

Egg Yolk Custard (Heavy Cream, Vanilla & Sea Salt)

Ingredients:

- 6 egg yolks
- 2 cups heavy cream
- 1 tsp vanilla extract
- A pinch of sea salt
- 1 tbsp sweetener (optional)

Instructions:

1. In a saucepan, heat the heavy cream over medium heat, but don't let it boil.
2. In a separate bowl, whisk the egg yolks, vanilla, and salt (add sweetener if using).
3. Slowly pour the hot cream into the egg mixture, whisking constantly.
4. Pour the custard mixture back into the saucepan and cook on low heat, stirring until thickened (about 5-7 minutes).
5. Remove from heat and cool before serving.

Note on bone broth: Unless you're making your own bone broth, remember to buy brands that use only wholesome ingredients; *Kettle & Fire*, and *Kitchen Basics* are good examples.

Chapter 6: Carnivore Kitchen Mastery: Recipes, Tips, and Techniques

Imagine waking up each morning with a clear plan, knowing exactly what nourishing meals await you. Like having a personal chef, minus the fancy apron. As you embark on this carnivore journey, you'll find that simplicity is not only your friend but also your secret weapon. The first week (after the 6-week transition) sets the tone, gently guiding you into the rhythm of a meat-centric lifestyle. You'll discover that the magic of the carnivore diet lies in its straightforward approach. No need for complex recipes or a pantry full of exotic ingredients. Instead, you'll focus on the pure, unadulterated goodness of nutrient-dense proteins and fats.

In this inaugural week, we strip away the clutter, honing in on what truly nourishes you. Forget about lengthy ingredient lists and obscure spices. The beauty of carnivore meals is their simplicity. You're left with only the best—the nutrient-packed core of your diet. You're getting back to basics and enjoying the rich, savory flavors that nature intended. Think of it as a culinary detox, where you eliminate the unnecessary and embrace the essentials. With each meal, you'll fuel your body with high-quality proteins and fats that offer a wealth of benefits, from muscle repair to sustained energy.

As you ease into this new way of eating, remember that hydration and electrolyte balance are crucial. Transitioning to a carnivore diet can alter how your body processes minerals, so staying hydrated is more important than ever.

Mindful eating is another key component of your carnivore journey. In our fast-paced world, meals often become just another task to tick off the list. But there's so much more to savor when you slow down and truly engage with your food. Take a moment to appreciate the aroma of a sizzling steak, the texture of a juicy burger patty, the taste of well-seasoned meat. This practice not only enhances your dining experience but also helps you listen to your body's hunger and fullness cues. By focusing on the sensory elements of your meals, you cultivate a deeper connection to what you're eating and why.

Mindful Eating Checklist

Pause Before You Eat: Take a deep breath and check in with your hunger levels.

Engage Your Senses: Notice the colors, textures, and aromas of your food.

Chew Thoroughly: Savor each bite and chew slowly to aid digestion.

Reflect on Satisfaction: After your meal, reflect on how it made you feel physically and emotionally.

This first week is about laying a solid foundation. You're not just changing what you eat; you're transforming your relationship with food. By focusing on simple, satisfying meals and embracing mindful eating practices, you set yourself up for a successful transition into the carnivore lifestyle. Welcome to a new chapter of well-being.

Mastering a few basics can elevate your meals when it comes to cooking techniques. Searing meats in a cast-iron skillet enhances flavor and boosts your food's iron levels. The intense heat locks in juices, creating a beautiful crust that adds depth of flavor. Similarly, roasting techniques can be your best friend. They're perfect for bringing out the best in meats, ensuring optimal flavor with minimal fuss. These skills aren't just about getting through this week; they're tools you'll use again and again, building confidence in the kitchen as you explore new recipes and ideas.

Time-saving tips can make your culinary life smoother. Consider taking a little time to do some meal prep, say over the weekend, to pre-slice meats, or taking meat from the freezer to the refrigerator to thaw over a couple of days. This way, they're ready when you need them, cutting down on prep time. Batch-cooking meats is another great time-saver. Grill or roast a larger quantity than you'll eat in one sitting and store the extras. Having cooked meats on hand means you can assemble meals quickly. These small habits add up, making meal preparation less of a chore and more of an enjoyable routine.

Nutrient density is the name of the game, especially as you adapt to the carnivore lifestyle. Optional organ meats, such as liver, are nutritional powerhouses, rich in vitamins A, B12, and iron. If you're hesitant about the taste, sneak small portions of them into your meals. Chop finely and mix with ground beef for burgers or meatballs. This way, you get all the benefits without overwhelming your palate. Remember, this week is about setting a strong foundation, focusing on meals that nourish your body while keeping things simple and enjoyable.

Incorporating Variety and Culinary Techniques

As you move into the second week of your carnivore experience, it's time to add a little flair to your meals. You've got the basics down, and now it's the perfect time to experiment with different cooking methods that bring out the best in your proteins. Slow-cooking is a fantastic way to achieve tenderness that melts in your mouth, ideal for those tougher cuts of meat like brisket, chuck, or shoulder. Imagine the rich aroma of a slow-cooked pot roast wafting through your home, the meat tender enough to cut with a fork. It's a simple technique that transforms everyday ingredients into something extraordinary.

Smoking meats is another method that introduces a depth of flavor that's hard to resist. Like a rack of ribs with a smoky finish, the kind that has everyone asking for seconds. Smoking isn't just about flavor; it creates an experience. The process infuses your meats with a unique character, enhancing the natural flavors without overpowering them.

If you're looking for a precise approach, consider sous vide cooking. This technique involves vacuum-sealing your meat and immersing it in a water bath at a controlled temperature. It ensures your steak is cooked perfectly medium-rare, juicy, and tender every time, without the guesswork. I use the *Anova Precision Cooker Pro* (often on sale). If you don't have a vacuum sealer, no problem; I personally use *Swoofe* brand resealable silicone bags (available at Amazon) – just use the displacement method of removing air from the bag. Lower the open bag of meat into the water, allowing the water to force the air out of the bag, then zip it closed. If the bag doesn't stay completely submerged, you'll need to weigh it down with something; a sealed jar of water works great. Once you try sous vide cooking, and discover that you can have tender, but still medium-rare meats, you'll be hooked. There's a reason 5-star restaurants use it.

Variety in protein sources adds excitement and nutritional benefits. Lamb chops and pork belly offer rich flavors and textures distinct from beef or chicken. Lamb, with its subtle earthiness, pairs beautifully with herbs like rosemary and thyme, while pork belly delivers a savory richness that's unparalleled. Then there's the world of game meats, such as venison, which offer a lean yet flavorful alternative. These proteins diversify your diet and keep your meals interesting.

Seasoning is another arena where you can unleash your creativity. Herbs like rosemary, thyme, and sage can elevate a simple dish, adding layers of complexity. Explore different types of salts—like smoked salt—to bring out the natural flavors of your meats. Balancing these elements can turn a basic ingredient into a gourmet experience. Don't hesitate to experiment with marinades, either. A simple marinade of olive oil, garlic, lemon juice, and herbs can transform a cut of meat, creating new and exciting flavor profiles.

Encouraging creativity in the kitchen means personalizing your recipes. This could be as simple as adding a splash of lemon juice to brighten a dish or trying out different spice combinations to see what pairs well with your favorite cuts. The kitchen is your playground, and there's no right or wrong way to explore it. Experimenting keeps your meals fresh and helps you discover new tastes and preferences. As you try different techniques and flavors, you'll find what resonates with you, making your carnivore meals not just a dietary choice but a culinary adventure.

Building Confidence and Routine

As you step into the third week, confidence in your carnivore lifestyle begins to take root. Developing consistent habits is key to maintaining this momentum. Start with a regular shopping schedule. Knowing when you'll restock your pantry each week removes the guesswork, ensuring you always have what you need at your fingertips. Create a weekly menu in advance, mapping out each meal so you're not caught off guard. This not only streamlines your routine but also frees up mental space for other pursuits. Having a plan in place means less stress and more focus on enjoying the process and the meals themselves.

This week is also about giving yourself permission to experiment and adapt recipes to better suit your tastes. If you find a dish a little too spicy, adjust the seasoning to hit that sweet spot just for you. Or perhaps you've been sticking to beef and chicken—why not switch things up with pork or seafood? Substituting protein sources can keep your meals exciting and ensure your taste buds never get bored. The carnivore diet doesn't have to be rigid; let it flex with your preferences. This adaptability makes it easier to stick with long-term, turning it from a diet into a lifestyle.

Keeping the diet engaging helps to sustain motivation. Trying new recipes weekly can introduce fresh flavors and techniques into your culinary repertoire. Think of it as a mini-adventure for your palate. Joining cooking challenges, perhaps through online communities or social media groups, can also provide a fun and supportive way to test your skills and creativity. These challenges often come with themes or specific ingredients, pushing you to think outside the box and discover new favorites. Trying something new can reignite your enthusiasm and keep the journey enjoyable. There are endless carnivore or keto recipes in online blogs, social media groups, and videos.

Tips, Techniques, & Meat Temperature Guides

Even seasoned cooks encounter hiccups, so having some tips at your disposal can save the day.

- Avoiding overcooking is a common concern; it can turn a juicy steak into a dry disappointment. Pay attention to cooking times and internal temperatures appropriate for each cut of meat. An instant-read meat thermometer is invaluable here, ensuring that your meals are perfectly cooked every time.
- Beef Internal Temperature Guidelines:
  Rare: 125°F (52°C)
  Medium-Rare: 135°F (57°C)
  Medium: 145°F (63°C)
  Medium-Well: 150°F (66°C)
  Well-Done: 160°F (71°C) and above
- Poultry Internal Temperature Guidelines:
  Chicken: 165°F (74°C)
  Turkey: 165°F (74°C) for the breast,
  175°F (80°C) for the thigh
- Pork Internal Temperature Guidelines:
  Pork Tenderloin: 145°F (63°C)
  Pork Loin: 145°F (63°C)
  Pork Shoulder (Pulled Pork): 195°F (91°C)
- Different cuts require different cooking methods, times, and temps, so be open to adjusting your approach.
- Wet brining flavors and tenderizes meat by immersing it in a solution of salt, maybe some sugar-free sweetener, water, and various aromatic spices. The meat is submerged in the liquid brine and placed in the refrigerator for a specified period, allowing it to absorb flavors and moisture. This technique is particularly effective for poultry and lean cuts of meat.
- Dry brining, a method of seasoning and enhancing the flavor of meat by rubbing it with a mixture of salt and sometimes other dry

seasonings, is particularly popular for larger cuts of meat like roasts and whole poultry. Just rub it onto the meat, and refrigerate for a period of time.

- Marinating is a culinary technique where meat or seafood is soaked in a liquid mixture known as a marinade, which typically uses a combination of liquids, acids, oils, herbs, spices, and seasonings. The primary purpose of marinating is to infuse the food with flavor, enhance its tenderness, and sometimes contribute to its preservation.
- Resting meat for 5-10 minutes after cooking ensures optimal juiciness, allowing the juices to redistribute throughout the meat. It's a simple step, but it makes a big difference in the final dish.
- Achieving the perfect sear is another skill worth mastering. Use a hot iron skillet and let the meat form a natural crust without constant turning. This creates a beautiful caramelized exterior while keeping the inside tender and juicy.

These techniques are the foundation of restaurant-quality dishes, bringing professional flair to your home kitchen, and reinforcing your confidence. The more you practice, the more intuitive it becomes. You'll find that with each meal, your ability to navigate the nuances of carnivore cooking grows, turning each dish into a satisfying and rewarding experience. As these skills solidify, meal preparation becomes less of a task and more of an enjoyable ritual, one that nourishes both body and soul.

Additional Recipe Resources

On the days where you're not very hungry for lunch, but feel like you want just a little something, consider a simple beef broth[48] – homemade or store-bought. It's not just about warming your soul; it's about nourishment. Broth is a powerhouse of minerals that support your body's electrolyte needs, especially important as you adjust to this new diet. Bone broth is also rich in collagen, supporting joint health and digestion. Prepare a large batch over the weekend and store it in the fridge. You can reheat a portion whenever you need a quick, nutritious pick-me-up – be sure to scoop some of the solidified beef tallow along with the broth before heating, and add sea salt to taste. This approach not only saves time but also ensures you have a healthy option ready at your fingertips. Many people reuse the bones to flavor other soups before tossing them.

At the link below you will find a multitude of recipes, many of which are make-ahead carnivore-friendly casseroles, like…

Breakfast Casserole, Carnivore Quiche, and Carnivore Mac 'N Cheese

https://peopleschoicebeefjerky.com/blogs/news/carnivore-diet-recipes?srsltid=AfmBOoptUtPNx5rqVB6YN2AfPJ1C-T79YdvJ1Sn6LFuy91RGoLlLub9x

Rachel Elizabeth offers a simple carnivore recipe for…

Homemade Bone Broth:

https://www.ribeyerach.com/post/carnivore-diet-bone-broth-recipe-simple-easy

Oven-roasted chicken thighs are the perfect comfort food for dinner. They're juicy, flavorful, and incredibly satisfying, as simple as they are delightful, and allow the natural flavors of the chicken to shine through. Plus, chicken thighs are rich in B vitamins and zinc, supporting your immune system and energy metabolism.

Here's a recipe from ThePrimal.com:

Chicken Thighs

https://www.theprimal.com/carnivore-diet-recipes/carnivore-chicken-thigh-recipe-with-only-two-ingredients

We're diving into the world of diverse cuts and flavors, where every meal becomes an opportunity to explore culinary creativity. Let's start with bone-in beef short ribs (bone-in means they are true beef ribs; boneless usually means chuck), a dish that transforms a humble cut into a rich, succulent delight.

Here's a recipe for slow-cooker short ribs from TheStayAtHomeChef.com:

Slow Cooker Beef Short Ribs

https://thestayathomechef.com/slow-cooker-beef-short-ribs/

Next up, herb-roasted lamb chops offer a sophisticated twist with minimal effort. The herbs create a fragrant crust that complements the lamb's natural richness. The simplicity of this dish belies its elegance, making it great for both casual meals and special occasions. The combination of fresh herbs and tender lamb elevates the dining experience, proving that you don't need complex techniques to create a standout meal.

Here's a recipe from Anna Vocino:

Herb-Crusted Lamb Chops

https://annavocino.substack.com/p/herb-roasted-lamb-chops?utm_source=publication-search

Enhancing flavors can be as simple as adding a touch of garlic butter to your steak. Melt some butter with minced garlic and a sprinkle of parsley, then drizzle it over your cooked steak. The warm, buttery goodness enriches the meat's natural taste, adding a luxurious finish. Similarly, a hint of lemon zest on grilled fish can brighten the dish, adding a refreshing contrast to the savory flavors. These simple additions can transform a simple meal into something extraordinary, showing that sometimes, less truly is more when it comes to flavor.

International influences can spice up your carnivore repertoire. Imagine Korean BBQ-style beef, a tender, flavorful dish that's both exotic and familiar.

Here's a recipe from OliviaWyles.com:

Korean BBQ-Style Beef

https://oliviawyles.com/keto-korean-beef/#recipe

Or elevate your weeknight with a time-saving, simple but perfectly-seasoned pork roast[49]. Roasted to perfection, this dish embodies rustic charm, proving that a carnivore diet can still offer a world of flavors.

Here's a recipe for seasoned pork roast from GirlCarnivore.com:

Seasoned Pork Roast

https://girlcarnivore.com/oven-roasted-pork-tenderloin/

Quick and Easy for Busy Days

Life can get hectic, and when it does, quick and easy recipes can be a real lifesaver.

Here's a recipe for a tasty beef stir-fry, ready in just 20-minutes, from CarbManager.com:

Beef Stir-Fry

https://www.carbmanager.com/recipe-detail/ug:7f71007b962145e98a915ac103dfab8a/animal-based-beef-steak-stir-fry

The internet is full of wonderful carnivore (and keto) recipes, free of charge, to ignite creativity in the kitchen. You can reinvent the wheel if that's your thing; or you can keep it simple and copy the wheel. 😉

The following list, and many more, can be found at

Main Dishes, Snacks, Make-Ahead, & More.

https://carnivore.diet/carnivore-recipes/

MAIN DISHES:

PKD Adapted Shepherd's Pie Recipe
Carnivore Egg-in-a-Hole Recipe
Mozzarella-Stuffed Meatballs
Carnivore Stroganoff Recipe with Ground Beef
Carnivore Breakfast Muffins
Carnivore Casserole with Ground Beef (Breakfast or Dinner)
Carnivore Meatballs (Zero Carb)
Carnivore Salad
Organ Meat Pie
Carnivore Meatballs with Beef Heart
3-Ingredient Carnivore Scotch Eggs (No Pork)
Crustless Mini Meat Pies (with Hidden Liver)
Creamy Cheese Soup
Rotten Eggs (not really rotten, a different take on deviled eggs)
Cornbread (made with chicken, eggs, and butter)
Italian Meatballs
Cream Cheese Crepes

Philly Cheesesteak
Eggs Benedict
Meatza Pizza
Your Favorite Stuffed Burger
Spicy Chicken Cheesy Muffins Recipe
Cheeseburger Casserole
Cobb Salad
Meat Waffles
Chicken Taco Soup
Loaded Scrambled Eggs
Breakfast Casserole

SNACKS:

Bacon Cheese Chip Snacks
Pemmican
Grass-Fed Beef Liver Chips
Carnivore Snax Mix
Pepperoni Chips
Breakfast Pizza
Cheesy Flatbread
Your Favorite Cheese Crisps
How to Make a Beautiful Charcuterie Board

MAKE AHEAD:

Chili Stew (a great make-ahead meal)
Cream of Chicken Soup

CONDIMENTS:

Hollandaise Sauce
Beef or chicken liver pate with bacon
Keto Chicken Liver Pate

DESSERTS:

Carnivore Cake Recipe

Carnivore Egg Pudding Recipe
Egg Nog

And, if you're anything like me, you just can't give up on mayonnaise, which adds creamy moisture to any dish, but we don't want to those consume pesky seed oils, which contribute to inflammation. Following are some easy recipes to make this staple at home.

Homemade Classic Mayo (my own go-to recipe):

3/4 cup extra light tasting organic olive oil
1 whole egg (+ optional extra yolk if you happen to have one)
1/2 teaspoon sea salt
1 teaspoon lemon juice
1 teaspoon white vinegar
1/4 teaspoon mustard

Place all ingredients in a wide-mouth jar.

Lower immersion blender into jar over the egg. Blend about 20 seconds, and…Voilà! You have mayonnaise.

Carnivore Mayo (made with duck fat)

From Ash Eats

https://ash-eats.com/carnivore-mayonnaise-recipe/

Butter Mayo

From Cooking Keto With Lee

https://cookingketowithlee.com/butter-mayo/

Bacon Mayo

From This Mom's Menu
https://www.thismomsmenu.com/bacon-mayo/

Efficient Meal Prep for Busy Schedules

Batch cooking is another strategy to keep in your culinary toolkit. By preparing large quantities, you ensure that you have ready-to-eat meals whenever you need them. Take roasts, for instance. Cook a large roast on the weekend and use it in different dishes throughout the week. Slice it thin for snacks or enjoy it as a main dish. This approach not only saves time but also ensures that you're consistently eating well, even on the busiest days. Plus, having a stockpile of home-cooked meals means you're less likely to resort to takeout, keeping you aligned with your health goals.

Following are some videos to help you get into the groove of batch-cooking.

7 Days of Carnivore Diet Meals in 2 Hours: Is It Feasible?

By Yegor Tarnakin

https://youtu.be/jfh2fIqiJ0k?si=jj_OJGTSh6uYUGd6

SCAN ME

Carnivore diet meal prep for weight loss. It's working!

By Jen at Delighted to Meat You

https://youtu.be/4wpqxebCK7s?si=Cx_rkY-U3XhGlasK

SCAN ME

2+ Weeks' Worth of LION DIET Meal Prep // Carnivore Diet

by Neah at Neah's Way

https://youtu.be/-42EluCecho?si=V4MqclcKDNK5yGxC

SCAN ME

Mastering Meal Prep and Planning

As you venture further into the carnivore lifestyle, organization becomes your best ally. Efficient meal prep planning not only saves time, it sets you up for success. Creating a meal prep checklist is a practical first step. Jot down the proteins you'll need for the week, the cooking methods you plan to use, and any necessary prep work like marinating or chopping. This checklist acts as your roadmap, ensuring you have everything you need at your fingertips. Pair this with a weekly meal planner, where you can map out breakfasts, lunches, and dinners. Seeing your meals laid out visually helps reduce decision fatigue and makes grocery shopping a breeze. It also allows you to spot gaps or redundancies in your menu, ensuring satisfying meals.

Delving into advanced meal prep techniques can further streamline your kitchen time. Rotating proteins is a clever way to maintain variety without overcomplicating things. For instance, cook a large roast on Sunday, enjoy it as a main dish, then use the leftovers in various ways throughout the week. This not only saves time but also keeps your meals interesting. Pre-marinating meats is another strategy that enhances flavor and tenderness. Prepare marinades in bulk—think olive oil, garlic, and herbs—and let your meats soak overnight in the refrigerator. This simple step infuses them with flavor, reducing cooking time and enhancing taste. When you're ready to cook, your marinated meats will be bursting with flavor, making mealtime a treat rather than a chore.

Storage and preservation methods are crucial in keeping your meals fresh and flavorful. Vacuum sealing is a game-changer for long-term storage. It removes air, preventing freezer burn, and preserving the quality of your meats for months, and easy to drop into a sous vide bath for cooking. If vacuum sealing isn't an option, zip-top freezer bags with the air squeezed out will Do. Airtight containers work wonders for keeping your cuts fresh. For day-to-day use, glass containers are your best bet. They're not only durable and reusable, but they also make reheating a cinch. Glass locks in flavors and moisture, ensuring that your meals taste just as good the second time around. Plus, seeing your dishes through the glass can be a motivating reminder of the delicious, healthy meals you've prepared.

As you refine your meal prep skills, taking time for self-assessment and reflection is invaluable. Reflect on the dietary benefits you've experienced—perhaps more energy, improved digestion, or fat loss. Acknowledge any challenges you've faced, whether it's adjusting to new flavors or managing social situations. This reflection helps you make necessary dietary adjustments, like tweaking portion sizes or trying new cuts of meat, or preparing better for outings. It's a continuous learning process, and being open to change is key to sustaining this lifestyle. By regularly evaluating your progress, you can celebrate your successes and address any areas that need improvement, ensuring that your carnivore journey is both rewarding and sustainable.

On a budget? No problem. Many people, this author included, have found that buying and eating only animal products, namely meat and fat, provided greater satiety for a longer period of time. This naturally reduces the volume of food consumed, and saves money overall. You're no longer buying carb-laden 'foods' and, even though you're actually spending more on meats than you were before, you'll probably find that your entire grocery bill is less.

13 Savvy Tips for the Carnivore Diet on a Budget

By Brian Bianchetti | People's Choice Beef Jerky

https://peopleschoicebeefjerky.com/blogs/news/carnivore-diet-on-a-budget?srsltid=AfmBOooaKWluVe3P3JvzFQzslFpAdZqcY5f3-ANu2t2jSai3k2loD5o1

SCAN ME

There's a certain peace that comes with having a plan, especially when it comes to your diet. As you settle into the carnivore lifestyle, long-term meal planning becomes your ally. Not just choosing what to eat, but crafting a routine, keeps you engaged and excited about your food. Variety is key here, and it's what keeps the monotony at bay. Rotating between different types of meats like beef, pork, poultry, and seafood can transform your meals from mundane to magnificent. Each type of meat brings its own unique flavor and texture to the table. By diversifying your protein sources, you ensure that you're keeping your taste buds interested.

Variety doesn't stop at the type of meat. Experimenting with new recipes on a regular basis can add a fresh twist to your culinary repertoire. Try a new cooking method or flavor profile each month to keep things fresh. Perhaps one month you master the art of slow-roasting a pork shoulder, while the next month involves perfecting a spicy Cajun-style shrimp dish. This approach not only keeps your meals exciting but also expands your cooking skills, turning meal preparation into an enjoyable and creative endeavor.

I had never even heard of flanken ribs, but I found some at Sam's Wholesale Club, and just had to try them. They're regular beef ribs, but sliced across, rather than in-between, the bones, about ½" - ¾" thick. A breeze to cook—just use your favorite seasoning rub, spread them out on a foil-lined cookie sheet, and bake at 350-degrees for one hour, turn and bake for an additional hour, then slather with your favorite sugar-free BBQ sauce, and bake at 450-degrees for 10 minutes, or place under the broiler, until bubbly and crispy.

Another way to maintain interest is through seasonal meal planning. Each season offers its own bounty of low-carb produce that can complement your carnivore meals beautifully (unless you're doing strict carnivore). In the spring, you might find yourself incorporating fresh asparagus or radishes into your dishes, while autumn could inspire the addition of roasted Brussels sprouts or sautéed mushrooms. These seasonal ingredients add a splash of color and flavor to your plate, enhancing your meals without straying from your dietary goals. Seasonal produce not only offers freshness but often aligns with your body's changing nutritional needs throughout the year.

For those who love a theme, themed meal nights can be a delightful addition to your routine. Imagine hosting an international cuisine night, where you explore flavors from around the world while staying true to your carnivore principles. One week, you might indulge in a Brazilian BBQ night, featuring skewered meats and flavorful marinades. The next, you could journey to the Mediterranean with a feast of lamb chops and olives. These themed nights provide a sense of adventure and discovery, making mealtime an experience rather than just a necessity.

Planning efficiency is the backbone of sustaining this lifestyle long-term. Utilizing tools like weekly meal planning templates can save you time and stress by streamlining the process. These templates allow you to map out your meals for the week, ensuring you have all the ingredients you need and preventing last-minute trips to the grocery store. Additionally, apps for recipe storage and meal tracking can be invaluable. They offer a convenient way to organize your favorite recipes, track your dietary progress, and make adjustments as needed. With these tools at your disposal, meal planning becomes a seamless part of your routine, freeing up time for other pursuits and helping you stay committed to your goals.

Action Step: Weekly Meal Planning Template

Consider using a simple meal planning template for each day of the week. To keep things simple, we have one available for you as a free bonus (see Bonus section). It even includes a list of meats and seasoning herbs. Use this template to guide your shopping list, ensuring you have everything you need for a successful week of carnivore eating.

Embracing variety, seasonal produce, and creative themes keeps your meals exciting and aligned with your carnivore lifestyle. It's about finding joy in the process and making meal planning an enjoyable part of your routine. As you continue this journey, remember that sustaining the carnivore lifestyle is not just about what you eat but how you approach your meals with intention and enthusiasm.

The Economics of Eating Carnivore: Budgeting and Sourcing

Navigating the financial end of the carnivore lifestyle doesn't have to be daunting. We have found that after ditching higher carb unfulfilling foods and concentrating on meats and fats, we actually spend less money than before carnivore. With a few clever strategies, you can save even more while enjoying high-quality meals. One of the best ways to save money is by buying in bulk from wholesalers. Think about it—purchasing larger quantities of meat reduces the price per pound, and you can always freeze what you don't eat immediately. Sharing the cost with a like-minded friend is also an option. This approach not only slashes costs but also ensures you have a variety of meats at your disposal. Local farmers' markets are another goldmine for fresh, affordable options. By cutting out the middleman, you often find better prices and get to know the folks who raise your food. Plus, the quality is typically top-notch, which is exactly what you want when you're fueling your body with nutrient-dense foods.

Choosing the highest-quality meat you can afford is worthwhile. Grass-fed meats tend to have higher omega-3 fatty acid content, less omega-6, and more antioxidants, which can be a boon for your health. However, they also come with a higher price tag. However, grain-fed meats offer a more affordable choice without sacrificing much in terms of nutritional value. For those who prefer the convenience of online shopping, meat subscription services deliver quality cuts straight to your doorstep. These services often offer a variety of options, from pasture-raised beef to wild-caught seafood, allowing you to choose what best suits your needs and budget.

Building relationships with local suppliers can yield more than just cost savings. By joining community-supported agriculture (CSA) programs, you gain access to fresh, seasonal produce and meats directly from the farm. These programs often offer bulk buying options, which means more savings in your pocket. Visiting local farms is another way to source high-quality meats while supporting your community. Many farms offer the chance to buy meat directly, sometimes at a discount, especially if you purchase in larger quantities. Knowing the origin of your food and the practices behind its production fosters a deeper connection to what you consume.

The websites below can help to find local farm suppliers:

Eat Wild

https://eatwild.com/

SCAN ME

Local Harvest

https://www.localharvest.org/

SCAN ME

USDA Local Food Portal

https://www.usdalocalfoodportal.com/

SCAN ME

Market Wagon

https://shop.marketwagon.com/shop

SCAN ME

Financial planning can be an integral part of maintaining the carnivore diet without overspending. Start by creating a monthly food budget that aligns with your dietary goals. This budget acts as a roadmap, helping you prioritize essential purchases and avoid unnecessary expenses. Tracking expenses with financial apps can further streamline this process, offering insights into spending habits and highlighting areas where you can cut back. It's surprising how much you can save when you eliminate junk food and focus on high-quality meats. Not only does this approach enhance satiety, meaning you eat less overall, but it also results in spending less on fillers that don't contribute to your health goals.

Budget Tips:

- Budget-Friendly Shopping Checklist
- Buy in bulk from wholesalers or warehouse stores.
- Visit local farmers' markets for fresh, affordable options.
- Consider grain-fed meats for a budget-friendly alternative.
- Explore online meat subscription services for convenience.
- Join CSA programs or visit local farms for direct sourcing.
- Create a monthly food budget and track expenses with apps.

Embrace the economics of the carnivore diet by focusing on quality over quantity; remember that a little planning goes a long way. By implementing these strategies, you can enjoy the benefits of the carnivore lifestyle without feeling the pinch in your wallet.

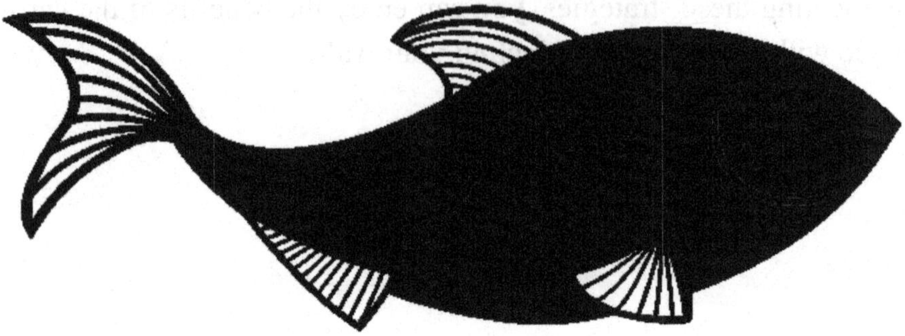

WHEN & WHERE

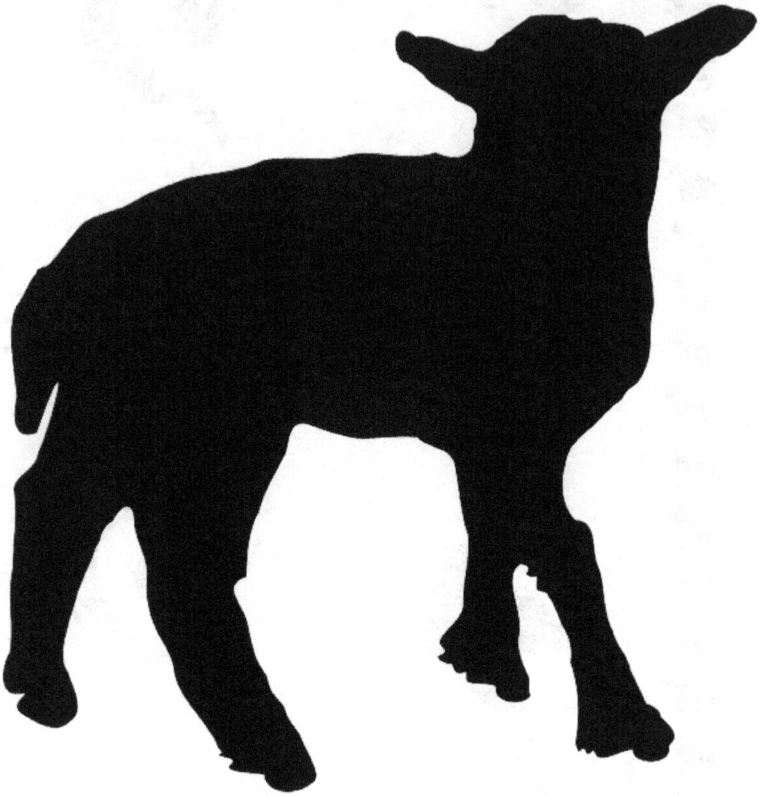

Chapter 7: Beyond the Plate: Lifestyle Integration

Enjoy Carnivore With Your Family

Integrating a carnivore diet with family meals might seem like a balancing act at first, but with a few thoughtful strategies, you can create meals that satisfy everyone at the table. The key is versatility. Preparing dishes that can easily adapt to various preferences is a game-changer. Picture a hearty platter of grilled meats, where each family member can choose their favorite cut or seasoning. This approach not only satisfies diverse tastes but also simplifies meal planning. Gone are the days of pleading with picky eaters to finish their greens; instead, you can focus on dishes that everyone enjoys. It's liberating to watch your family savor meals without the usual dinnertime negotiations over vegetables.

Children can be the toughest critics, so having a few kid-friendly carnivore recipes up your sleeve is a must. Mini meatballs with a variety of dipping sauces offer both fun and flavor. Imagine a plate of juicy meatballs paired with homemade ketchup[50] or a creamy cheese dip. The bite-sized portions are perfect for little hands and make mealtime interactive and enjoyable. Savory egg muffins are another hit. Packed with protein, these muffins can be customized with different fillings, like bacon or cheese, to keep things interesting. They're easy to make and perfect for breakfast or a snack, ensuring your kids get the nutrients they need without fuss. They also travel well!

It's natural to have concerns about meeting your children's dietary needs. Rest assured, a carnivore diet provides the essentials. Meat and fat are nutrient-dense, supplying vital vitamins and minerals crucial for growth and development. Ensure that your kids consume beef to cover their nutritional bases; after that, they can choose to eat a variety of other meats if they wish. While fruits and vegetables are often associated with vitamins, meats offer complete nutrition, including heme iron and vitamin B12 which cannot be found in any plant foods. Focusing on quality cuts and incorporating optional organ meats occasionally can further enhance their diet, making sure they're getting everything they need to thrive.

Family involvement in meal planning and cooking can transform your kitchen into a space full of creativity and connection. Organize family carnivore cooking nights where everyone can pitch in. Let your kids choose a recipe, gather ingredients, and help with preparation. This involvement not only teaches valuable cooking skills but also fosters a sense of ownership and excitement about meals. You could even turn grocery shopping into an adventure, encouraging your children to pick out cuts of meat or explore new flavors. When kids feel included in the process, they're more excited about the meals, more likely to eat them, and more likely to develop a positive relationship with food.

Balancing a carnivore diet with family life doesn't mean sacrificing variety or enjoyment. It's about making thoughtful choices that accommodate everyone's needs while simplifying the cooking process. By focusing on versatile, nutrient-rich meals and encouraging family participation, you create a dining experience that's both nourishing and harmonious. Your table becomes a place where everyone looks forward to sharing meals and memories, surrounded by the delicious simplicity of a carnivore lifestyle. Much like our ancient ancestors enjoying the fruits of the day's hunt around the campfire.

Handling Holidays and Special Occasions with Ease

Holidays and special occasions can be a minefield of dietary temptations. They are often centered around food, and it's easy to feel dismayed by the array if options don't fit your carnivore lifestyle. But planning is your ally here. Start by prioritizing protein-rich dishes at gatherings. Whether it's a holiday feast or a backyard barbecue, focus on the meats. Think a juicy steak, turkey, or ham. These options not only align with your diet but also keep you satiated. You can even contribute a dish, ensuring there's something you can enjoy without concern. A platter of grilled meats or a selection of charcuterie can be both a crowd-pleaser and a diet-saver.

Celebrations don't have to mean straying from your dietary goals. Imagine serving an herb-crusted prime rib, perfectly seasoned and roasted to perfection. It's a dish that screams special occasion without deviating from your carnivore principles. The herbs add a burst of flavor, while the tender meat satisfies your holiday cravings. If you're looking for something a bit more casual, consider bacon-wrapped appetizers. They're easy to make and incredibly versatile. Wrap slices of bacon around shrimp, chicken bites, or little smoked sausages, bake until crispy, and watch them disappear from the platter. These dishes not only keep you on track but also showcase the delicious potential of a carnivore feast.

Social pressures can be tricky to navigate. It's common to face questions or critiques about your dietary choices during these events. Prepare yourself with a few thoughtful responses. When someone asks, "Why aren't you having dessert?" you might reply, "I'm focusing on my health and this way of eating works best for me." Keeping your explanations simple and personal often diffuses curiosity without turning into a debate. If someone persists, you can always steer the conversation towards the benefits you've experienced, like increased energy or better digestion. "I have so much more energy since ditching sugars in favor of nutrient dense foods!" Sharing your positive results can be more persuasive than any scientific explanation.

While it's important to stay committed, holidays are also about enjoyment and connection. Encourage yourself to indulge mindfully. This doesn't mean throwing your diet out the window, but rather, setting personal boundaries that allow for flexibility. Perhaps you decide that indulging at your favorite Chinese buffet once every two to three months is your treat. This approach helps you enjoy life's moments without feeling guilty. It's about finding a balance that honors your health goals while allowing you to partake in social rituals. Remember, one meal won't undo all your progress. It's the consistent choices that matter the most.

Incorporating these strategies can make it more pleasant to approach holidays and special occasions. With a bit of forethought and flexibility, you can enjoy these events without compromising your dietary commitments. It becomes less about what you can't have and more about celebrating what you can—delicious, satisfying meals that support your health and well-being.

Practical Strategies for Social Situations and Dining Out

Navigating social events and dining out while sticking to the carnivore diet might seem daunting at first, but it's entirely doable with a little preparation and creativity. When eating out, focus on meat-centric dishes. Most restaurants offer various meat options, whether a juicy steak, roasted chicken, or a grilled seafood platter. Don't hesitate to customize your order. Request that your meat be cooked in butter instead of oils, and ask for extra servings of meat or eggs in place of the usual sides like bread or potatoes. This approach not only keeps you on track but often leads to discovering delicious new combinations that align with your dietary needs.

Hosting gatherings can be a strategic way to maintain control over your food options. Planning a carnivore-friendly menu ensures you have plenty to enjoy while also introducing your guests to the delights of meat-based dishes. Consider a grill-out where you can showcase a variety of meats—think sausages, ribs, and burgers. Adding a few simple sides, like cheese platters or deviled eggs, caters to all preferences. Hosting these events not only allows you to stick to your dietary goals but also creates an opportunity to share your enthusiasm and knowledge about the carnivore lifestyle with others.

When it comes to alcohol and non-meat options, you'll want to make informed choices. If you choose to drink alcohol, opt for low-carb options such as dry wines, or spirits like vodka and whiskey, which can be enjoyed without mixers. These options typically have minimal impact on your carbohydrate intake, as long you limit your servings to one or two. For non-meat foods, consider low-carb options like leafy greens or a small cheese board if you feel inclined. These choices can complement your meal without taking you off track. Being mindful of your selections allows you to participate in social events without straying from your carnivore principles.

Sticking to the carnivore diet while navigating social settings and dining out requires a bit of strategy and flexibility. By focusing on meat-centric options, preparing for social interactions, and making thoughtful choices, you can enjoy these experiences without compromising your health goals. With practice, these strategies become second nature, helping you balance your dietary commitments and your social life.

Carnivoring on Planes, Trains, and Automobiles

Traveling while sticking to a carnivore diet might sound like a challenge, but with a bit of planning, you can stay on track without compromising your health goals.

Here are some practical and carnivore-friendly ideas for packing travel foods that cater to the whole family, regardless of the mode of transportation:

General Packing Tips

- **Use Insulated Bags or Coolers**: Keep perishable items fresh, especially for road trips. Consider ice packs or frozen gel packs that comply with travel regulations.
- **Portion Control**: Pack individual servings to make it easier to distribute snacks and meals, especially for kids.
- **Compact Containers**: Use lightweight, spill-proof containers to save space and prevent messes.
- **Prep Finger Foods**: Foods that don't require utensils are easier to handle while traveling.

Car-Friendly Foods

- **Hard-Boiled Eggs**: Easy to eat, nutrient-dense, and satisfying. Peel them in advance for convenience.

- **Cheese Sticks or Cubes**: Great for kids and adults alike. Keep them cool in a small insulated bag.
- **Meat Roll-Ups**: Roll deli meat (e.g., turkey or roast beef) around cheese or cream cheese for a filling snack.
- **Cooked Bacon or Sausage Links**: Delicious cold or at room temperature.
- **Jerky or Meat Sticks**: Opt for sugar-free, nitrate-free versions if possible.

Plane Travel Tips

Since liquids and gels are restricted, focus on solid, non-perishable options:

- **Vacuum-Sealed Meats**: Pack mini sealed foil packs of tuna, chicken, or salmon. Bring a travel fork for easy access.
- **Biltong or Air-Dried Meats**: Similar to jerky but often more tender and flavorful.
- **Hard Cheeses**: Cheese like Parmesan or Gouda doesn't require refrigeration for short trips.
- **Cooked Chicken Strips**: Boneless and easy to eat, these work well for meals or snacks.
- **Packaged Pork Rinds**: A crunchy, mess-free snack alternative to chips.

Train and Bus Ideas

For longer journeys, focus on foods that are easy to store and eat without much fuss:

- **Cold Cuts and Charcuterie**: Combine sliced meats with olives or pickles for a simple, handheld meal.
- **Mini Meatballs**: Make a batch of bite-sized meatballs ahead of time and eat them cold or at room temperature.
- **Deviled Eggs**: Mix yolks with mayo and spices for a filling (make sure the filling is more solid for planes). Use a small, secure container.

- **Smoked Salmon or Trout**: Pack thinly sliced smoked fish with a few lemon wedges.
- **Pre-Cooked Burger Patties**: Stack patties with cheese between parchment paper for easy transport.

Kid-Friendly Options

- **Meat-and-Cheese Skewers**: Use toothpicks to create fun, bite-sized snacks.
- **Chicken Nuggets (Carnivore Style)**: Make homemade nuggets with pork rind breading for a healthier option.
- **Ham and Cheese Roll-Ups**: Simple, mess-free, and tasty.
- **Egg Muffins**: Packable and customizable with family-favorite flavors.

Travel Meal Packs

Prepare compact meals for long trips:

- **Carnivore Bento Boxes**: Pack cooked meats, hard cheeses, boiled eggs, and olives in a divided container.
- **Salmon Salad Wraps**: Wrap salmon salad in thin slices of meat instead of a tortilla.
- **Mini Frittatas**: Make ahead in muffin tins and fill with meats and cheese.

Navigating airport food options can be tricky, but it's not impossible. Many airports now offer a range of dining choices, including restaurants that serve grilled meats or omelets. In fact, one of the best meals I've ever had was slow roasted beef brisket at the airport in Charlotte NC. If you're in a rush, opt for hard-boiled eggs or cheese from a deli counter. These simple choices can keep you satisfied during layovers or delays. On long flights, staying committed to your diet requires a bit more planning. Pack a small cooler with boiled or deviled eggs, liver pate, cooked bacon strips, or even cook a few steaks in advance to enjoy mid-flight. Not only does this keep you on track, but it also saves you from the often expensive and less-than-ideal food options available at airports.

Portable meal solutions are a traveler's best friend. Homemade beef jerky is ideal—not only is it protein-packed, but it's also lightweight and non-perishable. Canned sardines are another excellent travel companion. They're compact, full of healthy omega-3s, and easy to pop open whenever hunger strikes. Dehydrated meat chips offer a crunchy alternative, adding variety to your travel snacking. These options ensure you have a reliable source of energy and nutrition, no matter where your adventures take you.

If you're on the road…there are some restaurants beginning to buck the conventional scaremongering about saturated fats, ditching seed oils, and have gone back to using beef tallow for fried foods. Buffalo Wild Wings and Outback Steakhouse are a couple of those. Check out LocalFats.com to find restaurants in your area[51] using healthy fats.

The link below offers more carnivore travel tips from nutritionist Judy Cho. There's also a refreshing carnivore food pyramid, tips on car travel, snacks, and eating out.

Travel Hacks: Nutrition With Judy

https://www.nutritionwithjudy.com/travel-hacks-for-the-carnivore-diet#:~:text=To%20stay%20consistent%20with%20the,enhance%20flavor%20and%20nutrient%20intake

SCAN ME

By incorporating these ideas, you'll have plenty of variety to satisfy the whole family while staying aligned with carnivore principles.

Fueling Fitness with the Power of Carnivore

Stepping into the world of fitness while embracing a carnivore diet might seem like venturing into uncharted territory, but in reality, it's a natural pairing that complements your health journey. Imagine waking up, feeling the energy coursing through your veins, ready to tackle whatever the day throws your way. That's the power of aligning your nutrition with your fitness goals. Whether you're lifting weights, practicing yoga, or simply trying to stay active, the carnivore diet can enhance your performance and recovery in ways that might surprise you.

Strengthen Muscles and Protect Bones

With regards to building muscle, the carnivore diet offers a significant advantage. Protein is the building block of muscle, and with a meat-based diet, you're getting an abundance of high-quality amino acids that fuel muscle protein synthesis. This means that your muscles repair and grow more efficiently after a workout. The anti-inflammatory properties of a carnivore diet also play a role here, reducing recovery time and allowing you to hit the gym without feeling worn out. It's like having a secret weapon that keeps you on your toes, ready for the next challenge.

Protein is also a building block for healthy bones; about 50% of our bones, by volume, consists of protein. And, as we age, we need even more protein to maintain healthy muscles and bones.

Did you know that medications to build your bone density, and make them appear strong and white on a Dexa scan, can actually make your bones brittle and at greater risk of fracture? According to Dr. Mercola, *"Bisphosphonates will disrupt your body's bone-building process, resulting in the preservation of "old bone" rather than promoting healthy bone formation through natural methods."*[52] Scary, huh? It is nice to know that the carnivore diet and proper exercise can truly improve your bone health, not just make them appear stronger on a scan.

To calculate your personal protein needs, weigh yourself, then subtract the estimated pounds of excess fat; now you have an approximate number for your lean body mass. Aim to eat .5 to 1 gram of protein per pound of lean body mass, or 1-2 grams per kilogram of lean body mass, depending upon your level of activity. If you're a couch potato, go for the minimum; if you are very active, go for the upper number. A moderately-active 160-pound minus 20 pounds of excess fat has approximately 140 pounds of lean mass. She can strive for about 100 grams of protein daily (140 x .7, the middle of the range of .5 to 1 gram).

This provides your muscles and bones with the necessary fuel to grow and adapt. For endurance athletes, fat adaptation becomes critical. By training your body to use fat as its primary energy source, as the carnivore diet naturally does, you enhance your stamina and eliminate reliance on quick-burning carbs. This shift can lead to sustained energy levels during long runs or cycling sessions, allowing you to perform at your best.

Meanwhile, yoga practitioners might find unexpected improvements in flexibility. The diet's anti-inflammatory effects can ease joint discomfort, making transitions between poses smoother and more comfortable. It's about finding the synergy between what you eat and how you move, creating a holistic approach to health and fitness.

Strength-Training & Carnivore: A Dynamic Duo

Those involved in strength training will notice enhancements thanks to the protein intake that supports muscle growth and recovery, without having to overcome the hindrance of antinutrients. <u>And for those who aren't involved in strength-training, you should begin now. The carnivore diet, and the simple time-saving tweak below, offer amazing benefits for muscle, bone, and overall quality of life. Strong muscles effect strong bones and prevent osteopenia and osteoporosis.</u>

Pushing heavy weights, and focusing on the negative movement—like slowly lowering the weights after an arm curl—can maximize your workout efficiency, even allowing for an intense, full-body workout in under 30 minutes. Kevin and I work out this way, and people at the gym take notice. Strangers will often ask us about our routine. So after verbalizing—and Kevin loves to verbalize 😉—if he can tell they are genuinely interested in learning more, we offer them a sheet of paper to help them better absorb and retain the information. We have turned that sheet of paper into an ebook, *"Carefree Carnivore Workout & Eating Plan;"* showing how you can put forth maximum effort, and reap maximum reward, in minimal time at the gym. It is yours for the asking; see the Bonus section to get your free copy.

When it comes to workout nutrition, the carnivore diet offers some unique strategies. Since carnivore allows one to feel satiated for a much longer period of time, going through your workout on an empty stomach is not only doable, it's ideal. This is so the body can use all its energy for your workout without having to devote a good portion of energy to digestion. If glucose is needed to push through your workout, your body can create glucose as needed through gluconeogenesis[53]. However, if you find yourself hungry or weak prior to a workout (especially in the beginning of your carnivore experience), and feel you are under stress, a small meal rich in protein and fat can help, like bone broth and beef jerky, or a couple of deviled eggs. These are also great for post-workout recovery; rich in amino acids and electrolytes, these options help replenish your body and support muscle repair without added sugars.

Fitness Integration Checklist

- **Set Clear Fitness Goals:** Define what you aim to achieve—be it muscle gain, endurance, or general fitness.
- **Track Protein Intake:** Ensure you're getting enough protein to support your workouts.
- **Incorporate Varied Exercise Routines:** Mix strength training with flexibility exercises like yoga.
- **Optimize Pre- and Post-Workout Nutrition:** Choose meals that support your energy needs and recovery.

Integrating your carnivore diet with your fitness routine isn't just about eating more meat but understanding how this way of eating can support your specific goals and enhance your overall performance. Whether you're a dedicated athlete or someone who simply enjoys staying active, embracing these principles can transform the way you approach fitness, making it a more rewarding and effective part of your lifestyle.

Biohacking and Carnivore: Enhancing Performance and Health

Biohacking is all about taking control of your biology to achieve better health and performance. It's like being the pilot of your own health journey, steering your body toward optimal functioning. When you combine biohacking with a carnivore diet, you tap into a powerful synergy. The focus shifts to using diet as a tool to influence genetic expression. By nourishing your body with nutrient-dense foods, you're not just feeding yourself; you're unlocking potential at a cellular level. This approach can improve cognitive function, offering clarity and focus like never before. Imagine starting your day with a clear mind, ready to tackle complex tasks with ease. That's the magic of aligning biohacking with the carnivore lifestyle.

When it comes to practical biohacking methods, you have a toolbox full of options. Intermittent fasting stands out as a favorite among biohackers. Following are a couple of options for healthy people (be sure to read the Stress Management section later in this chapter). By restricting your eating window, you give your body a chance to reset and rejuvenate. This practice can enhance metabolic health, promote fat loss, and even improve mental clarity. It's like giving your body a mini-vacation, letting it focus on repair and maintenance instead of constant digestion. Another intriguing method is cold exposure. Whether through a cold shower or an icy plunge, this technique can boost resilience, increase energy levels, and even improve mood. It's a wake-up call for your system, invigorating your body and mind.

Experts in the biohacking community offer valuable insights that can guide your journey. Dave Asprey , a pioneer in the field, often highlights the benefits of nutrient-dense foods, emphasizing their role in cognitive enhancement and overall well-being. His work suggests that what you eat directly impacts how you perform, both mentally and physically. Biohacking is a journey of self-discovery, where the goal is to unlock your full potential.

The outcomes of biohacking can be both tangible and transformative. Many people report an improvement in mental clarity and focus, finding themselves more productive and capable of tackling complex tasks. It's as if a fog lifts, revealing a clearer path forward. Improved sleep quality is another common benefit. By aligning your diet and lifestyle with your body's natural rhythms, you enhance your ability to rest and recharge. This leads to better energy levels during the day, making it easier to stay active and engaged. Biohacking isn't just about quick fixes; it's about creating sustainable changes that support long-term health and vitality.

Stress Management: Supporting Your Journey

Stress. It's something we all face, and while a little stress can push us to meet deadlines or prep for big events, chronic stress is a different beast. It can derail our best-laid plans, including dietary goals. Imagine trying to stick to your carnivore diet when you're stressed out—it's like trying to build a sandcastle in a storm. Stress affects everything from digestion to nutrient absorption, so managing it is crucial. When you're stressed, your body might not absorb the nutrients from your meals as efficiently, impacting your energy levels and overall well-being. You might find yourself reaching for comfort foods, veering off your dietary path. Reducing stress isn't just about feeling better; it's about making sure the diet you're committed to actually works in your favor. Dr Izabella Wentz explains it all very well in her "Adrenal Transformation Protocol," and offers a natural and simple approach to addressing the effects of chronic stress .

Enter adaptogens, nature's little helpers. These are natural substances that can help your body handle stress more effectively. Rhodiola is one of those adaptogens known for its remarkable effects on energy levels. It can help you feel more alert during the day and manage stress without the jittery side effects of caffeine. Another noteworthy adaptogen is Ashwagandha, an herb that has been shown to reduce cortisol levels—the stress hormone that can create havoc in your body when elevated for too long. Lowering cortisol not only calms your mind but also supports your body's ability to burn fat and maintain muscle. Including adaptogens in your routine can provide a subtle yet significant boost, helping you manage stress.

There are simple, practical strategies you can incorporate into your daily life to tackle stress head-on. Try mindful breathing exercises; they can be done anywhere, anytime. Focus on your breath for just a few minutes, and you'll notice a calming effect that steadies your mind. Meditation is another powerful tool. Even a short, five-minute session can help clear your mind and reduce anxiety.

If you're looking for something a bit different, consider alternating hot and cold water in your shower. Switch between temperatures for 15-second intervals, repeating for two to three cycles. This practice can stimulate your adrenals, providing either a calming effect for overactive systems or a boost for sluggish ones.

Stress management isn't just about feeling zen; it will help you stick to your dietary goals with more ease. When stress is under control, your digestion improves, and your body absorbs nutrients more effectively. This means your meals do more for you, supporting your energy and health.

Interestingly, consuming animal fat can also help reduce stress by providing a source of steady energy and nutrients that support brain health and mood stability. Wake up in the night and can't go back to sleep? Eat a tablespoon of grass-fed butter. Incorporating healthy fats can make your meals not only satisfying but also calming. It's like giving your body a resourceful ally that helps you face daily challenges with a bit more resilience.

Understanding how stress impacts your diet and taking active steps to manage it can transform your experience with the carnivore lifestyle. It's not just about the food; it's about creating a balanced life where your diet, stress levels, and overall health align seamlessly. By integrating adaptogens and stress-reduction techniques, you can enhance your ability to stick to your carnivore diet and enjoy its benefits more fully.

Adapt Gradually For Long-Term Success

When embracing the carnivore diet, it's tempting to dive in headfirst, expecting immediate changes. But like any significant lifestyle shift, gradual adaptation is key. Allowing your body to acclimate at its own pace can make all the difference in achieving long-term success. Think of it as training for a marathon rather than a sprint. Your body needs time to adjust, to learn how to efficiently process this new way of eating. It's not just about swapping foods; it's about teaching your metabolism a new rhythm. This slow and steady approach helps minimize initial discomfort, like the common "keto flu" symptoms, while setting a sustainable foundation for the future.

It can be challenging to stay motivated over time, especially when the initial excitement wanes. One effective strategy is setting long-term health goals. These goals act as a guiding light, reminding you of the bigger picture beyond daily fluctuations. Whether it's increased energy, improved skin, or better digestion, having clear objectives keeps you focused. Regularly revisiting your personal motivation is also crucial. Reflect on why you started this journey in the first place. Was it to feel more vibrant? To manage a chronic condition? Reminding yourself of these reasons can reignite your passion and commitment, providing the fuel needed to keep going. This is where keeping a journal of goals, moods, and symptoms along the way can be invaluable.

Food Lists, Journals, Assessment

Below is a simple and useful document which includes a before- and after-assessment, food lists and journals, and even a food reintroduction journal, from Precision Nutrition: https://assets.precisionnutrition.com/2021/04/the-smart-carnivore-diet-plan.pdf

Adaptation isn't always smooth sailing. Plateaus can test your patience, but they're a natural part of the process. When progress stalls, it's an opportunity to reassess and make tweaks. Maybe it's time to explore different cuts of meat or adjust your meal timing. Lifestyle changes can also pose challenges. Social gatherings, work events, or travel might require creative solutions to stay on track. Flexibility is your ally here. Being prepared with options helps you navigate these situations without feeling derailed. Remember, adaptation is about evolving with the flow, not resisting it.

The carnivore diet isn't static; it evolves with you. Incorporating new recipes and techniques keeps things fresh and exciting. Perhaps try sous vide cooking for perfectly tender meat or experiment with different herbs and spices to elevate flavors. Learning and adapting as you go fosters a deeper connection to the lifestyle, making it a dynamic journey rather than a rigid routine. This mindset encourages exploration and curiosity, transforming challenges into opportunities for growth. It's about finding joy in the process and celebrating progress, no matter how small.

As you continue adapting to the carnivore diet, remember that sustainability comes from flexibility and resilience. Embracing the path with an open mind and a willingness to learn not only supports your health goals but also enriches your overall experience. Real change takes time, but with patience and persistence, the rewards are well worth it. You've set the stage for a fulfilling lifestyle, where food supports your vitality and well-being.

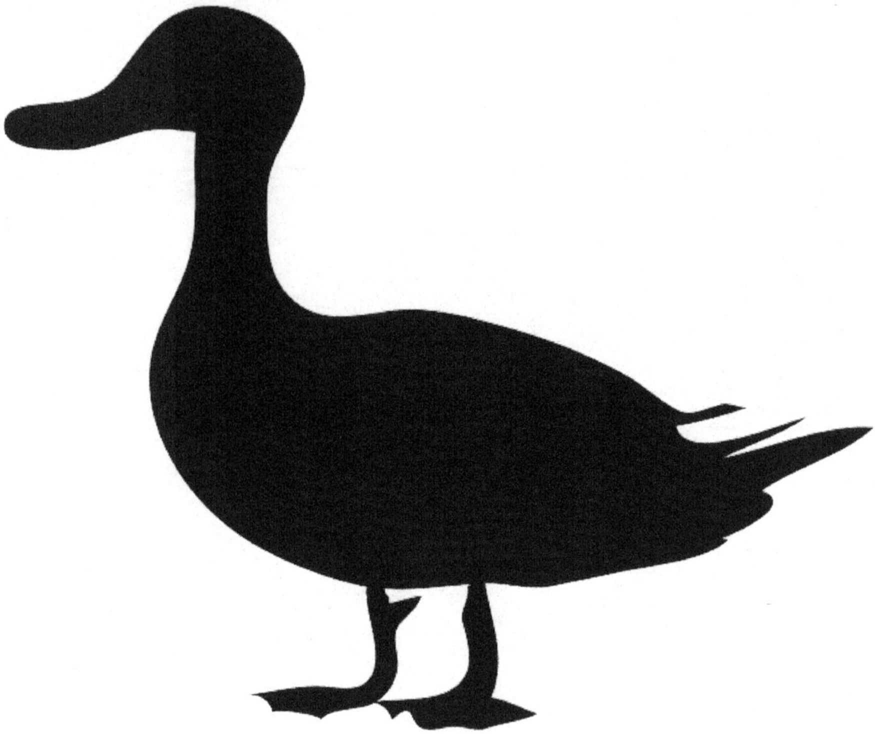

Chapter 8: Sustaining the Carnivore Lifestyle

Reintroducing Foods on the Carnivore Diet

After you've settled into the carnivore lifestyle and experienced the benefits, you might start thinking about reintroducing non-carnivore foods. You don't have to; you can survive, and thrive, on carnivore indefinitely—just like our ancient human ancestors did. However, if you decide to reintroduce foods, It's a step that requires a careful approach, with the understanding that your newfound well-being will suffer to some degree. After all, if you go back to eating the way you were before carnivore, it won't take long for your old health problems to resurface, excess fat creeps back on, and the joint pain returns.

To reintroduce foods, start with foods that are low in allergens and carbohydrates. These types of foods are generally easier on the system and less likely to trigger adverse reactions. Think of starting with something like a small serving of leafy greens or a bit of avocado. As you try these foods, pay close attention to how your body reacts. Your energy levels, digestion, and overall mood can provide vital clues about how well you're tolerating these additions.

Reintroducing foods is a bit like conducting an experiment, and with any experiment, you want to watch for potential pitfalls. Some foods might trigger symptoms that you hadn't anticipated. Identifying and avoiding these so-called trigger foods is crucial. These could manifest as bloating, fatigue, or even skin flare-ups. By keeping a keen eye on your body's responses, you can pinpoint which foods support your health and which ones might need to be removed from your diet again. This process isn't about rushing; it's about finding a balance that allows you to enjoy a varied diet without sacrificing the benefits you've gained from the carnivore approach.

Mindful experimentation is key here. Introduce one food at a time, wait several days to a week before introducing another. Consider keeping a detailed food diary as you introduce foods back into your diet. This diary acts as a logbook, helping you track not only what you eat but also how you feel afterward. Documenting your meals and any symptoms that arise can help you establish patterns and make informed decisions about your diet. Was it the dairy in your coffee that caused the bloating, or was it the handful of almonds you snacked on? A well-maintained food diary can provide these answers and guide your future dietary choices.

There are several structured plans available to guide your reintroduction process, each tailored to different dietary experiments. For instance, when it comes to dairy, start with fermented options like yogurt or kefir, which tend to be easier on digestion. Gradually work your way up to harder cheeses. If vegetables are on your list, begin with those that are low in carbohydrates, lectins and oxalates, such as zucchini or cucumbers minus the seeds. These are less likely to disrupt digestion and can be a gentle way to expand your palate.

Nutritionist Judy Cho offers some guidance:

How to Reintroduce Food On Carnivore Diet | Nutrition with Judy

https://www.nutritionwithjudy.com/how-to-reintroduce-food-on-a-carnivore-diet#:~:text=Begin%20by%20reintroducing%20one%20food,to%20monitor%20your%20body's%20reaction

SCAN ME

Whether you choose to incorporate more variety into your diet or prefer to stick closely to carnivore principles, the decision is yours. Listen to your body and let it guide you through this phase. Some people find that they feel so good on carnivore that they choose to keep it simple and enjoy their newfound health. Others appreciate having a bit more flexibility. Whatever you decide, remember that your journey is unique. The goal is to find a balance that keeps you feeling your best while allowing you to enjoy the foods you love.

Fine-Tuning Your Diet: Listening to Your Body's Needs

As you continue with the carnivore diet as your base, it becomes crucial to tune into your body's signals. Think of biofeedback as your body's way of communicating its needs, a kind of internal dialogue that guides your dietary decisions. Recognizing signs of nutrient deficiencies is part of this conversation. Perhaps after reintroducing some foods you notice a dip in energy or changes in skin health—these could be indicators that your body craves certain nutrients. Adjusting your macronutrient ratios based on how you feel is a way to respond. If energy levels are lagging, increasing your fat intake might provide the needed boost, while adding back some protein could enhance strength and recovery.

Personalization in diet is the secret sauce to long-term success. Just like how no two people have the same fingerprint, your nutritional needs are unique to you. Tailoring your protein and fat intake to match your lifestyle and health goals can make a world of difference. For instance, someone who engages in regular strength training might benefit from a higher protein ratio to support muscle growth, while another focused on endurance might thrive on an increased fat intake for sustained energy. This customization ensures that your diet works with your body, not against it, allowing you to thrive.

Tools for self-assessment play a vital role in this fine-tuning process. Regular check-ins with health professionals can provide insights that you might miss on your own. These visits offer an opportunity to discuss your progress, address any lingering concerns, and tweak your diet as needed. Health professionals, especially those in favor of the carnivore lifestyle, can offer advice grounded in science, and tailored to your specific circumstances. Alongside professional guidance, consider incorporating personal assessments into your routine. Are you feeling more energetic? Sleeping better? Tracking these changes helps you evaluate your diet's effectiveness and make informed adjustments.

Continuing education about your nutritional needs keeps you ahead of the curve. This ongoing learning is not just about keeping up with trends; it's about empowering yourself with knowledge that supports your well-being. Whether it's subscribing to a carnivore nutrition podcast or reading the latest articles, or watching the latest videos, integrating education into your lifestyle keeps nutrition at the forefront of your mind, and enhances your ability to make informed dietary decisions.

Self-Assessment Checklist

- Regularly evaluate energy levels and overall well-being.
- Track dietary changes and their effects on mood and performance.
- Consult with health professionals for personalized advice.
- Stay up to date with the latest carnivore expert insights.

Listening to your body is an art worth mastering. By interpreting its signals, personalizing your approach, and committing to ongoing education, you create a dynamic process that supports sustained health and vitality. This approach transforms your relationship with food from one of mere consumption to one of mindful nourishment, where every meal is an opportunity to support your body's needs. The beauty of this process lies in its adaptability, allowing you to respond to your body's cues and make informed choices that lead to a healthier, more balanced life.

Building a Support Network: Engaging with Online and Local Communities

As you deepen your commitment to the carnivore lifestyle, finding a community that shares your values can be incredibly rewarding, as mentioned in Chapter 4. Being part of a supportive group can make all the difference, providing emotional encouragement and practical advice that smooths out the rough edges of dietary shifts. Picture this: you've had a long day, and all you want is to connect with someone who gets it. In these moments, turning to a community of like-minded individuals can provide not just companionship but also a wealth of shared knowledge. This network becomes a space to share recipes, tips, and even troubleshooting advice for when things don't go as planned. It's where you can learn from others' experiences and celebrate your own successes, knowing you're not alone on this path.

Finding and joining these groups is easier than ever, thanks to the digital age. Social media platforms are buzzing with carnivore-friendly forums and groups, each filled with individuals at various stages of their personal transformations. These online spaces offer real-time interaction, allowing you to ask questions and get a variety of answers from people who've walked the same road. Local meetups and workshops provide an opportunity for face-to-face connection, fostering friendships and offering a sense of belonging. Meeting others who share your dietary preferences can turn an isolating experience into one of kinship and understanding. These gatherings are often informal, allowing for relaxed conversation and the chance to swap stories over a shared meal.

Being part of a community is more than just receiving support; it's about active participation. Sharing your personal experiences and advice can enrich the group, offering insights that might help someone else overcome a challenge you've faced. By contributing, you not only solidify your understanding of the lifestyle but also inspire others who might be struggling or just starting out. Engaging in discussions, posing questions, and providing feedback all contribute to a vibrant and dynamic community.

Your involvement can create ripples, encouraging others to share their journeys and building a supportive environment.

Mentorship is another powerful aspect of community engagement. Learning from those who have spent more time navigating the carnivore lifestyle can accelerate your own progress. These seasoned veterans offer invaluable perspectives and guidance, helping you avoid common pitfalls, refining your approach. Consider reaching out to someone whose journey resonates with you. Ask questions, seek advice, and absorb the wisdom they've gained through experience. Conversely, as you become more comfortable and knowledgeable, you might find yourself in a position to offer mentorship. Sharing your learnings and helping newcomers find their footing can be incredibly fulfilling. It's a chance to give back to the community that supported you, creating a cycle of growth and encouragement.

Whether you're engaging online or in person, remember that the strength of a community lies in its diversity and shared purpose. Each member brings unique insights and experiences, contributing to the expanse of knowledge and support. Being part of such a network reminds you that you're not alone in your dietary choices. Instead, you're part of a collective endeavor to live healthier, more vibrant lives through the carnivore lifestyle. This sense of belonging can be a powerful motivator, helping you stay committed and inspired as you continue to explore the benefits of this dietary approach.

Avoiding Burnout: Keeping the Experience Fresh and Exciting

In every long-term endeavor, especially one as personal as a dietary lifestyle, there's a chance you'll face moments of burnout. It's that sense of routine fatigue—a feeling that your meals have become mundane, and the motivation to meal prep isn't as strong as it once was. Recognizing these signs early can be crucial. Maybe you're finding your meals predictable, or the thought of prepping another batch of ground beef just doesn't excite you anymore. It's a natural part of the process and acknowledging it is the first step in rekindling that initial spark.

To breathe new life into your carnivore journey, consider shaking up your cooking techniques. If you've been pan-frying everything, try grilling or slow-cooking to bring out different flavors and textures. Exploring exotic meats or cuts, or different herbs and spices can also renew your interest. Have you ever tried bison or venison? They offer a distinct taste that could reignite your culinary curiosity. These changes don't have to be drastic, but introducing variety can significantly alter your dining experience. It's like giving your taste buds a mini-vacation without leaving the comfort of your kitchen.

Setting new challenges can be an effective way to keep your commitment strong. Participating in a carnivore challenge, whether it's a 30-day commitment or a new recipe every week, provides structure and a sense of achievement. These challenges can be personal or shared with a community for added motivation. They not only help break the monotony but also offer a goal to work towards, which can be incredibly motivating. Challenges eject you from your comfort zone and encourage you to explore new aspects of the carnivore lifestyle you might not have considered before.

Moreover, integrating self-care into your routine is paramount. While diet plays a significant role in overall well-being, balancing it with lifestyle choices ensures a holistic approach to health. Incorporating relaxation techniques can alleviate stress and enhance your overall experience. Whether it's practicing mindfulness, taking a walk in nature, or even indulging in a hobby, these activities can refresh your mind and body. Remember, self-care is more than just the physical; it's about nurturing your mental and emotional health as well. When you take time for yourself, you're better equipped to appreciate and enjoy your dietary choices.

As you navigate these waves of enthusiasm and challenge, keep in mind that every experience is an opportunity for growth. Explore new avenues within your dietary framework, and don't shy away from trying different approaches. Whether it's a new cut of meat, a cooking method, or setting a personal goal, these strategies can keep your carnivore lifestyle as vibrant and enjoyable as it was on day one. This process is a journey of discovery, continually changing, and adapting to meet your needs and passions.

Reflecting on Your Journey: Lessons Learned and Future Goals

Reflection is more than just looking back—it's also understanding your experiences and learning from them. Taking the time to jot down your thoughts in a journal can be incredibly insightful. It's a simple, powerful tool that allows you to document successes and challenges along your path. As you write, consider what has worked well for you and where you've faced hurdles. This process not only helps solidify what you've learned but also highlights areas for growth. By regularly reflecting on your journey, you become more aware of the changes and progress you've made, providing a solid foundation, and motivation, for future endeavors.

In recognizing key lessons and insights, you'll likely find that the carnivore lifestyle has taught you more than just what to eat. It's about personal growth and a deeper understanding of your body's needs and capabilities. You might notice an increased awareness of how food impacts your energy, mood, and overall health. This awareness is powerful; it equips you with the knowledge to make informed choices in keeping with your goals. As you reflect, consider how these insights have shaped your approach to eating and living. What dietary habits have you developed? What have you learned about your body's unique responses to different foods?

With these insights in mind, setting future dietary and health goals becomes an exciting opportunity. Whether you're aiming to maintain your current health status, tackle a chronic condition, or further enhance your energy levels, having clear objectives can guide your actions. Think about long-term ambitions that resonate with your vision for health and vitality. Perhaps you're looking to incorporate more physical activity, or maybe you're interested in exploring new culinary skills within the carnivore framework. Whatever your goals, ensure they are specific, achievable, and meaningful to you. This clarity helps keep you motivated and focused on what truly matters.

Celebrating milestones is an integral part of staying motivated on this path. Recognizing your achievements, even small ones, reinforces positive behavior and fuels your commitment to the lifestyle. Consider rewarding yourself when you reach significant dietary milestones. This could be as simple as treating yourself to a new kitchen gadget or enjoying a day dedicated to self-care activities you love. These rewards act as reminders of your progress and perseverance. They bring joy to the process and encourage you to continue striving for your health goals. By appreciating the journey, you maintain enthusiasm and a sense of purpose.

Reflecting on your dietary journey is an ongoing practice that nurtures growth and self-awareness. By journaling about your experiences, you gain clarity on what works for you and what doesn't. This understanding is the cornerstone of personal growth, guiding you as you set new goals and celebrate your achievements. Embrace the lessons you've learned, and let them inspire your next steps. As you continue to explore the carnivore lifestyle, remember that each day offers a new opportunity to learn, grow, and enjoy the path you're on.

Embracing the Carnivore Identity: Living and Loving the Lifestyle

The carnivore diet is more than just what you put on your plate; it becomes a part of who you are. It's fascinating how a dietary choice can weave itself into the fabric of your identity. You might find yourself taking pride in your commitment, feeling a sense of accomplishment as you fuel your body with nutrient-dense foods, embracing the strength that comes with making deliberate, health-focused choices. When you adopt a diet that aligns with your values and goals, it becomes a reflection of your personal journey towards wellness. It isn't just about sticking to a plan, but celebrating the empowerment that comes with taking control of your health and well-being.

A positive mindset is key to sustaining this lifestyle. Viewing the carnivore diet as a lifestyle, rather than a restriction, shifts the focus from what you can't have to the myriad benefits you gain. It's about celebrating the newfound energy, the clarity of mind, and the health improvements you experience. By focusing on these positives, you cultivate a mindset that finds joy in the abundance of what you can enjoy. This way of thinking transforms the diet from a list of "don'ts" into a vibrant celebration of "do's." It encourages you to savor every meal, knowing it's nourishing not just your body but also your spirit.

One of the most beautiful aspects of the carnivore lifestyle is the sense of belonging it fosters. Engaging with a community of like-minded individuals can be incredibly fulfilling. Not just swapping recipes or sharing tips, but forming genuine connections with people who understand your choices and share your enthusiasm. These relationships can offer support, camaraderie, and a sense of shared purpose, making the journey less solitary and more communal. Whether it's through online forums, local meetups, or social media groups, finding your tribe can enrich your experience and provide a network of support that uplifts and inspires.

Living and loving the carnivore lifestyle is more than just committing to a diet. It's about embracing a new way of living, one that aligns with your values and enhances your sense of self. As you continue on this path, remember that your journey is unique and personal. Celebrate the victories, learn from the challenges, and let your identity flourish in the process. The carnivore lifestyle is about more than food; it's about the life you build around it, one choice at a time. Your story is still unfolding, and each chapter adds depth to your journey.

Conclusion

As we wrap up this journey through the carnivore diet, let's take a moment to reflect on what we've covered together. My goal in writing this book was to arm you with the tools and confidence to dive into a diet that's both ancient and revolutionary. This guide was crafted to help you cut through the noise and conflicting information, giving you a clear path to follow. It's about empowering you to take control of your health and vitality, using a diet that aligns with our evolutionary roots. Whether your aim is to boost your energy, manage chronic illness, or shed some body fat, I hope you now feel equipped to make informed choices.

You now know What, Why, How, When & Where to carnivore, and how to integrate your new lifestyle seamlessly with family. Throughout our chapters, we explored the fascinating roots of the carnivore diet and how it aligns with our ancestral past. We tackled myths and misconceptions, showing that a meat-based diet is indeed nutrient-complete. We delved into the practical side of things, with meal plans, recipes, and tips to help you adapt smoothly. We also discussed how to handle social situations and maintain this lifestyle without feeling isolated. And of course, we addressed concerns about long-term health impacts, backed by expert insights and scientific studies.

So, what are the key takeaways from our time together? First, remember that simplicity is your ally. The carnivore diet strips away the complexities and inadequacies of modern eating, allowing you to focus on nutrient-dense foods that truly nourish. Second, listen to your body. It's a powerful communicator, and by paying attention to its signals, you can tailor your diet to suit your individual needs. Third, stay flexible. Life happens, and it's okay to enjoy the occasional treat or adapt your meals to fit social gatherings. These principles serve as your compass as you continue on this path.

Now, I encourage you to take action. Begin by setting clear, realistic goals for your carnivore journey. Whether you're just starting or refining your approach, having a vision will guide your decisions. Dive into the meal plans, experiment with the recipes, and don't be afraid to try new things. Engage with the supportive communities we've mentioned, both online and locally, sharing your experiences, asking questions, and offering encouragement to others. Remember, you're not alone in this journey. There's a vibrant community of like-minded individuals ready to support you every step of the way.

I want to express my heartfelt gratitude for choosing this book as your guide. Writing it has been a labor of love, driven by my passion for helping people lead healthier lives. Your journey is important to me, and I'm here to support you. If you ever feel stuck or need a boost, remember that this book is always here for you. Each page was written with empathy and understanding, acknowledging the challenges and triumphs that come with any lifestyle change. I know them, because I've lived them.

As you continue on this path, I encourage you to foster a sense of community. Share your successes and struggles, and be open to learning from others. This journey is richer when shared, and the friendships you build along the way can provide invaluable support and motivation. By connecting with others, you'll find there is vast knowledge and camaraderie waiting for you.

You can begin the sharing experience right now, by taking just a moment to leave a review for this book. Doing so enables others to find it so they can begin their own journey to better health. Just click the link below or scan the QR code. Thanks so much!

https://www.amazon.com/review/create-review/?channel=glance-detail&asin=1966942001&ie=UTF8

With Sincere Gratitude,

Marsha

FREE BONUSES

- **Carefree Carnivore Workout & Eating Plan**—Take your workout to the next level with this free ebook, teaching you how to "accentuate the negative," and stop wasting time in the gym.
- **Weekly Meal Planner**—Use this printable sheet to plan your meals ahead of time to stay ahead of meal monotony. Use it to guide your grocery shopping list. It contains a handy list of meats and seasonings for inspiration.
- **Weekly Check-In Journal**—Use this simple, printable sheet to keep track of symptoms, notes on how you are feeling, and your progress on your carnivore journey.

Just drop me an email: MarshaShepherdWhitt@gmail.com.

IMPORTANT: To make sure I receive your email request, please use the following subject: **CAREFREE CARNIVORE BONUSES**

NOTE: Your information will never be shared with anyone else, and will be strictly used to make sure the requested information, and any future updates, gets delivered to your inbox without the spam monsters interfering.

REFERENCES AND ENDNOTES

---

[1] The word "evolution" evokes the idea in many Christians that science purports that humans came from apes (it doesn't). Some will also tell you that the earth is 6,000 years old, not 4.5 billion. As a Christian myself, I prefer to recognize that God is way bigger than the neat little boxes we sometimes try to fit Him into. The book of Genesis doesn't detail *how* God created the heavens and the earth—or even how long it took; a 'day' to God is not the same as a day to us. Maybe what science calls the "Big Bang" was how He chose to create the universe. Authentic science and faith aren't enemies—they're both on a quest for truth. To me, science helps us glimpse the *how* of God's work, while faith reminds us of the *why.* Why limit a God who created everything? That's the beauty of it—we don't have to.

[2] *Leroy, F., et a,* "The Role of Meat in the Human Diet: Evolutionary Aspects and Nutritional Value." *National Library of Medicine, PubMed Central*, 15 Apr. 2023, https://pmc.ncbi.nlm.nih.gov/articles/PMC10105836/

[3] *Richards, M. P., and Trinkaus, E,.* "Isotopic Evidence for the Diets of European Neanderthals and Early Modern Humans." *National Library of Medicine, PubMed Central*, 11 Aug. 2009, https://pmc.ncbi.nlm.nih.gov/articles/PMC2752538/

[4] *Sheffield, Sydney, et al,* "Nutritional Importance of Animal-Sourced Foods in a Healthy Diet." *Frontiers in Nutrition*, 24 July 2024, https://www.frontiersin.org/journals/nutrition/articles/10.3389/fnut.2024.1424912/full

[5] *Larsen, Clark Spencer,* "Biological Changes in Human Populations with Agriculture." *Annual Review of Anthropology*, vol. 24, 1995, pp. 185–213. *JSTOR*, http://www.jstor.org/stable/2155935

[6] *Ovadia, Dr. Philip,* "Feed Your Heart: The Secrets to Staying off the Operating Table." *TEDxJeffersonU*, 31 Jan. 2024, https://www.youtube.com/watch?app=desktop&v=jEBHrF1PNt4&t=306s&ab_channel=TEDxTalks

[7] *Mburu, Dr. Nam,* "Ascorbic Acid: The Forgotten Competition with Glucose." *Insulean*, 4 Dec. 2018, https://www.insulean.co.uk/ascorbic-acid-glucose/

[8] *Wrona, Thomas,* "Fiber Myths and Truths: Do We Really Need Fiber?" *Doctor Kiltz*, updated 4 Dec. 2023, https://www.doctorkiltz.com/fiber-myth/

[9] *Ho, Kok-Sun et a,* "Stopping or reducing dietary fiber intake reduces constipation and its associated symptoms." *World journal of gastroenterology* vol. 18,33 (2012): 4593-6. doi:10.3748/wjg.v18.i33.4593, https://pmc.ncbi.nlm.nih.gov/articles/PMC3435786/

[10] *Gunnars, Kris,* "9 Important Functions of Protein in Your Body." *Healthline*, 9 Feb. 2023, https://www.healthline.com/nutrition/10-reasons-to-eat-more-protein#TOC_TITLE_HDR_12

[11] *Tondt, Justin et a,.* "Application of nutrient essentiality criteria to dietary carbohydrates." Nutrition research reviews vol. 33,2 (2020): 260-270, doi:10.1017/S0954422420000050, https://pubmed.ncbi.nlm.nih.gov/32102704/

[12] *Salamon, Maureen,* "Low-Carb Diet Helps Cut Blood Sugar Levels in People with Prediabetes." *Harvard Health*, 3 Jan. 2023, https://www.health.harvard.edu/blog/low-carb-diet-helps-cut-blood-sugar-levels-in-people-with-prediabetes-202301032869

[13] *Merriam Webster Dictionary*, "Gluconeogenesis," n.d., https://www.merriam-webster.com/dictionary/gluconeogenesis

[14] *Jonasson, L., et al,* "Advice to Follow a Low-Carbohydrate Diet Has a Favourable Impact on Low-Grade Inflammation in Type 2 Diabetes Compared with Advice to Follow a Low-Fat Diet." *National Library of Medicine, PubMed Central*, 20 Apr. 2014, https://pmc.ncbi.nlm.nih.gov/articles/PMC4025600/

[15] *Dr. Philip Ovadia, TEDxJeffersonU,*"Feed Your Heart: The Secrets to Staying Off the Operating Table," January 31, 2024, https://youtu.be/jEBHrF1PNt4?si=UJ0bSDt_KJg1BVP4

[16] *Teicholz, Nina,* "Don't Blame Sugar: Food Producers Profited from the Demonization of Fat." *The Seattle Times*, 4 Oct. 2016, https://www.seattletimes.com/opinion/dont-blame-sugar-food-producers-profited-from-the-demonization-of-fat/

[17] https://physicalculturestudy.com/2015/01/07/vilhjalmur-stefanssons-all-meat-diet-part-one/

[18] https://physicalculturestudy.com/2015/01/12/vilhjalmur-stefanssons-all-meat-diet-part-two/

[19] *Jennifer Chesak,* reviewed by Dominic D'agostino, PhD, "What is metabolic flexibility, and why is it important?" updated Jul 22 2024, https://www.levels.com/blog/what-is-metabolic-flexibility-and-why-is-it-important

[20] *Bret H. Goodpaster, Lauren M. Sparks*, Metabolic Flexibility in Health and Disease, Cell Metabolism, Volume 25, Issue 5, 2017, Pages 1027-1036, ISSN 1550-4131, https://doi.org/10.1016/j.cmet.2017.04.015 (https://www.sciencedirect.com/science/article/pii/S1550413117302206)

[21] *Veronika Larisova,* "Logical Fallacies of a Vegan Diet: Why you shouldn't feed a child a vegan diet," Updated: Jun 24, 2024 https://wearechief.com/en-us/blogs/articles/why-you-shouldnt-feed-a-child-a-vegan-diet?srsltid=AfmBOooBcbaachkw9-A19d87CPqfMJDntcQIVMPwyVJbEOflzA3qHunH

[22] "How do Carnivores get their nutrients?" Delighted to Meat You, YouTube, Marc 8 2023, https://youtu.be/rgjv1ohPz-A?si=Di-tt1Rnjuy6KD75

[23] *Dr Nam Mburu,* "ASCORBIC ACID | The Forgotten Competition with Glucose," December 4, 2018, https://www.insulean.co.uk/ascorbic-acid-glucose/

[24] *Nutrition With Judy,* The Importance of Electrolytes for the Carnivore Diet, February 28, 2024, https://www.nutritionwithjudy.com/the-importance-of-electrolytes-for-the-carnivore-diet

[25] Dr. Elizabeth Bright, "Why supplementing with Lugol's Iodine is Essential," n.d., https://www.elizbright.com/article-posts/why-supplementing-with-lugols-iodine-is-essential

[26] *Michael Friëdman, ND*, Restorative Medicine Digest, November 23, 2016, "Interview with Thyroid Expert and Speaker David Brownstein, MD," https://restorativemedicine.org/digest/interview-thyroid-expert-david-brownstein-md/

[27] "You NEED Cholesterol for these 7 Things (Is Cholesterol Bad?)" Dr Ken Berry, MD, YouTube, June 26 2022, Updated 2024, https://youtu.be/kRtljOrDFpw?si=Fctk_79j7xbODq5H

[28] Dr. Eric Berg, :Why Cholesterol is so Biologically Important – Cholesterol Function," YouTube, December 8 2019, https://youtu.be/kND-iQDrhKI?si=9yFdSSWZQK3UEbHX

[29] *Newsweek*, "Heart Surgeon on His 95% Carnivore Diet: 'You Don't Have to Fear Red Meat.'" 23 Oct. 2024, https://www.newsweek.com/heart-surgeon-carnivore-diet-dont-fear-meat-1973701

[30] *Journal of the American College of Cardiology*, "Saturated Fats and Health: A Reassessment and Proposal for Food-Based Recommendations: JACC State-of-the-Art Review." Aug. 2020, https://www.jacc.org/doi/10.1016/j.jacc.2020.05.077

[31] "The truth about high cholesterol," Dr. Paul Mason, YouTube, Low Carb Down Under, Nov 19, 2022, https://www.youtube.com/watch?v=rdgS3PuSuyg

[32] *Dr. Richard Maurer,* "Know Your TG:HDL Ratio – Triglyceride / HDL-cholesterol," The Blood Code, September 21 2016, https://thebloodcode.com/know-your-tghdl-ratio-triglyceride-hdl-cholesterol/#:~:text=TG:HDL%20is%20one%20of,so%20I%20still%20advise%20restraint.

[33] *Liam McAuliffe,* Carnivore Diet for Autoimmune Issues? How it Works," "Doctor Kiltz, February 22 2024, https://www.doctorkiltz.com/carnivore-diet-autoimmune/

[34] *Kathryn Kos, M.Ed,* NTP, "Carnivore and the Gut Microbiome: Dispelling Myths About Fiber and Probiotics," Carnivore Bar, December 5 2024, https://carnivorebar.com/blogs/carnivore-bar-blog/carnivore-and-the-gut-microbiome-dispelling-myths-about-fiber-and-probiotics

[35] *Nih.gov,* "NIH study shows how insulin stimulates fat cells to take in glucose," September 7, 2010, https://www.nih.gov/news-events/news-releases/nih-study-shows-how-insulin-stimulates-fat-cells-take-glucose

[36] *Professor Bart Kay, YouTube, Main Channel,* "In 5 Minutes Or Less – the Randle Cycle," 2023, https://youtu.be/Gqrc7kInnCU?si=5GyzU9gWWiptYwLG

[37] *Dr. Thomas Seyfried,* The Charlie Foundation, YouTube, June 29 2020, https://youtu.be/TD-b4fttTNE?si=vv0clhoVNe_xoScV

[38] *Tanne, Janice Hopkins,* "Financial ties common between US medical schools and drug companies." *BMJ : British Medical Journal* vol. 335,7624 (2007): 793. doi:10.1136/bmj.39370.485880.13, https://pmc.ncbi.nlm.nih.gov/articles/PMC2034715/#:~:text=Two%20thirds%20of%20the%20costs,medical%20device%20companies%2C%20they%20report.

[39] https://www.dukehealth.org/find-doctors-physicians/eric-c-westman-md-mhs?utm_source=chatgpt.com

[40] https://lowcarbcardiologist.com/about/

[41] *Dr. Ken Berry,* YouTube, KenBerryMD, "What REALLY Causes HEART DISEASE ??" https://youtu.be/G8EEdi1XWU8?si=_gZLS2wYGwR3yN_v

[42] *Dr. Paul Mason,* Ep. 43: Dr Paul Mason - Carnivore Diet & Optimal Health, Meat the Ultimate Podcast, October 6 2019, https://youtu.be/90rpGhMehZ4?si=8JhBUbLmT8PhaKE-
[43] Dr. Kiltz, "Find a Keto + Carnivore Friendly Provider," https://www.doctorkiltz.com/keto-carnivore-doctors/
[44] "How to heal a gallbladder: Ketosis and Autophagy," Dr. Annette Boxworth, November 4, 2018, https://bozmd.com/how-to-heal-a-gallbladder-ketosis-and-autophagy/
[45] *Desai, Mahesh S et al.*, "A Dietary Fiber-Deprived Gut Microbiota Degrades the Colonic Mucus Barrier and Enhances Pathogen Susceptibility." *Cell* vol. 167,5 (2016): 1339-1353.e21. doi:10.1016/j.cell.2016.10.043, https://pmc.ncbi.nlm.nih.gov/articles/PMC5131798/
[46] *Inbound Pursuit,* "Carnivore Diet For Inflammation: Does it Help or Hinder Inflammatory Response?" Inbound Pursuit, May 12, 2023, https://carnivoresnax.com/blogs/articles/carnivore-diet-for-inflammation?srsltid=AfmBOopLG6PktQgKwoiXKpH0m-gvgAeRJBf6UNARVSq5lSC9I1lluD5K#what-the-science-says-about-carnivore-diet-and-inflammation
[47] *Dr. Ken Berry,* "10 Things a Carnivore Diet can do for You [Easy & Affordable] 2024," KenBerryMD, YouTube, July 24 2023, https://youtu.be/9RNCh_EmMHo?si=Mo6Ob0uckNA8W0pY
[48] *Ribeye Rach,* "Carnivore Diet Bone Broth Recipe (Simple & Easy)." *Ribeye Rach*, Updated 6 July, https://www.ribeyerach.com/post/carnivore-diet-bone-broth-recipe-simple-easy
[49] *Kita,* "Oven Roasted Pork Tenderloin." *Girl Carnivore*, Updated 12 June 2024, https://girlcarnivore.com/oven-roasted-pork-tenderloin/
[50] *Arman Liew,* Sugar Free Ketchup, February 26, 2024, https://thebigmansworld.com/keto-ketchup-sugar-free/
[51] Find restaurants cooking with good fats, https://localfats.com/
[52] *Dr. Joseph Mercola,* This Silent Disease Affects Millions of Americans, November 02, 2024, https://media.mercola.com/ImageServer/Public/2024/November/PDF/osteoporosis-silent-disease-pdf.pdf
[53] "Gluconeogenesis," Merriam Webster Dictionary, n.d., https://www.merriam-webster.com/dictionary/gluconeogenesis

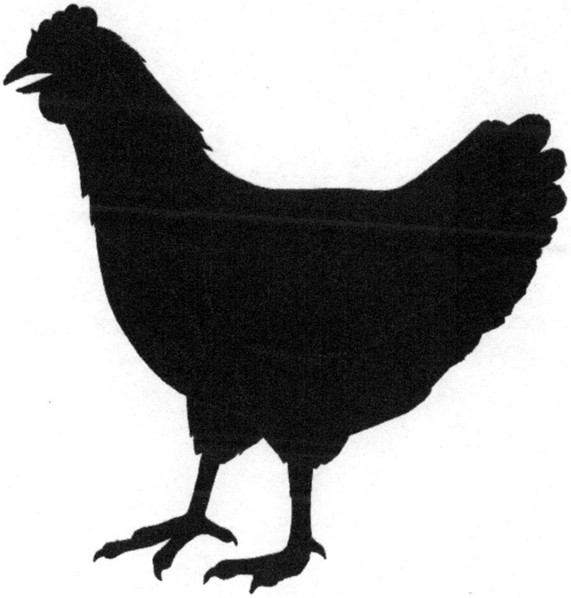

Made in the USA
Monee, IL
04 November 2026

67385782R00089